CONFIDENT CALCULATIONS

The Easy Guide to Drug Calculations for Student Nurses

Understand It. Calculate It. Check It. Decide Safely.

Dr Benjamin Olusola Ajibade
Ajibade Academic Publishing

Copyright and Edition Information

Confident Calculations: The Easy Guide to Drug Calculations for Student Nurses

First Edition.

Published by Ajibade Academic Publishing, Newcastle upon Tyne.

ISBN (Paperback): 978-1-919077-20-8

ISBN (Ebook): 978-1-919077-21-5

This edition has undergone nursing editorial review. Readers relying on this book professionally are encouraged to verify current clinical guidance directly against the primary sources listed in Further Reading and Resources, and against their own organisation's medicines policy, since clinical guidance is periodically updated and a printed book cannot update itself.

About the Author

Dr Benjamin Olusola Ajibade is an Assistant Professor in Mental Health Nursing at Northumbria University, and an Honorary Professor at SEETA University, Uganda. He holds a Professional Doctorate in Nursing, is a Senior Fellow of the Higher Education Academy, and is registered with the Nursing and Midwifery Council as both a nurse and a teacher.

His teaching and research focus on inclusive mental health and social care, with a particular interest in health inequalities affecting racially minoritised communities, and in methodological innovation, including the use of LEGO® Serious Play® to explore student transitions into higher education. He has published widely in nursing education and mental health practice, and has led national and international collaborations aimed at widening access to postgraduate research and improving the experience of students and staff from underrepresented backgrounds.

Confident Calculations grew directly out of his classroom experience: watching capable students freeze in front of drug calculation questions, not because they lacked mathematical ability, but because the subject is so often taught as a set of formulas to memorise rather than a way of reasoning to understand. He is the founder of ELEVATE, an initiative supporting early-career and minoritised researchers, and writes under the Ajibade Academic Publishing imprint.

You can find more of his work through his institutional profile at Northumbria University, or through the Ajibade Academic Publishing catalogue.

Disclaimer

This book is an educational resource intended to build understanding of the mathematical reasoning behind drug dose calculations. It is not a substitute for your employing organisation's medicines management policy, for the current British National Formulary or British National Formulary for Children, for manufacturer product information, or for the professional judgement of a prescriber or pharmacist.

Specific figures used as examples in this book, including drop factors, insulin concentrations, and maximum doses, are illustrative and intended to teach a calculation method. They are not a substitute for checking the actual figures printed on the medication, device, or prescription in front of you at the time of administration. Always verify current dosing information, local policy, and product-specific guidance before administering any medication.

Neither the author nor the publisher accepts liability for any loss, harm, or damage arising from reliance on the content of this book in place of current clinical guidance, local policy, or professional judgement.

Who This Book Is For

This book is written primarily for pre-registration nursing students working through drug calculation numeracy assessments, and for newly qualified nurses consolidating that learning into early clinical practice. It is equally useful as a refresher for experienced staff who want to rebuild genuine understanding underneath calculation habits developed over years of practice.

It assumes no more mathematical background than is covered in Part One of this book. It does assume you are working, or training to work, within a UK clinical and regulatory context, since specific figures, terminology, and regulatory references throughout reflect that setting.

A Note on NMC Alignment

The Nursing and Midwifery Council's Standards of Proficiency for Registered Nurses require accuracy in calculating and administering medicines as a core proficiency for registration. Nursing programmes approved against these standards require the medicines calculation component of numeracy assessment specifically to be passed at 100%, not a majority mark.

This book does not exist to add to the pressure that figure understandably creates. It exists because a requirement that strict deserves a learning approach built on genuine understanding rather than memorised shortcuts that fail under unfamiliar conditions. The full reference for this standard is included in Further Reading and Resources at the back of the book.

A Message to the Student Who Thinks They Can't Do Maths

If you have picked up this book already convinced that you are simply not a maths person, you are not alone, and Chapter 1 speaks to exactly that feeling directly. For now, here is the short version: most people who believe this about themselves are wrong about it, and the belief itself is doing more damage than any actual gap in ability. Read Chapter 1 before you decide this book isn't for you.

If, having read Chapter 1, you recognise something in yourself that sounds more like a specific numeracy learning need than anxiety, that is worth taking seriously and worth raising with your institution's learning support services. Either way, you are in the right place to start.

Acknowledgement

This edition was strengthened by independent editorial review covering clinical accuracy, medication safety guidance, and instructional design, alongside nursing editorial review. Ajibade Academic Publishing thanks the reviewers for the care taken in that process. Any remaining errors are the author's responsibility, and readers who identify one are encouraged to contact the publisher.

Contents

How to Use This Book 1

Before You Begin: Reading the Prescription Safely .. 3

PART I — Build the Foundations 6

Chapter 1: Why Drug Calculations Cause Anxiety (and How This Book Fixes That) 7

Chapter 2: Core Numeracy Refresher: Fractions, Decimals, Percentages, and Ratios 13

Chapter 3: Units and Conversions: The Silent Cause of Serious Errors 19

PART II — Master Everyday Doses 23

Chapter 4: Tablets and Capsules: The Core Method 24

Chapter 5: Liquid Medications and Oral Suspensions 30

Chapter 6: Practice Set 1: Tablets, Capsules, and Liquid Medications 35

PART III — Injections and High-Risk Medicines 38

Chapter 7: Calculating Injection Volumes 39

Chapter 8: Understanding Drug Concentrations: Units, Insulin, and Heparin 45

Chapter 9: Practice Set 2: Injections, Reconstitution, and Unit-Based Dosing 50

PART IV — Intravenous Calculations 53

Chapter 10: Calculating IV Flow Rates 54

Chapter 11: Infusion Time and Volume Calculations 59

Chapter 12: High-Risk IV Medications: Why These Need Extra Checks 63

Chapter 13: Practice Set 3: IV Flow Rates and High-Risk Infusions 67

PART V — Weight-Based and Paediatric Calculations 70

Chapter 14: Weight-Based Dose Calculations 71

Chapter 15: Body Surface Area Calculations 75

Chapter 16: Paediatric-Specific Safety Considerations....................79

Chapter 17: Practice Set 4: Weight-Based, BSA, and Paediatric Dosing...84

PART VI — Think, Check and Perform with Confidence...87

Chapter 18: Common Error Patterns and How to Catch Them Before They Reach the Patient...88

Chapter 19: Double-Checking Strategies That Actually Work....92

Chapter 20: Calculation Confidence Under Pressure......................96

Chapter 21: Mock Assessment: Final Challenge..............................100

Chapter 22: Mock Assessment: Foundation to Challenge.............103

Chapter 23: Mock Assessment: Comprehensive Review................106

Quick Reference Formula Sheet..109

Glossary..111

Further Reading and Resources...112

Solutions..117

How to Use This Book

This book is built to be worked through in order, not dipped into at random. It is organised into six parts, from core numeracy in Part I through to the confidence and checking habits in Part VI, and each part rests on the reasoning built in the one before it. The worked examples get harder to follow if the foundations underneath them are shaky, so if you are already confident with an earlier topic, read the chapter anyway, briefly, since the way ideas are framed here carries through to everything that follows.

Every teaching chapter follows the same shape: a plain explanation of the idea, worked examples with every step shown and justified, and a short set of key points at the end. Some chapters also include a Spot the Error box, presenting a flawed calculation for you to critique before seeing why it fails, and a Before You Calculate checklist to run through prior to working any clinical question.

Four Practice Sets, after Parts II, III, IV, and V, and a Mock Assessment near the end of Part VI, bring together everything covered up to that point in mixed questions, graded Foundation, Clinical Application, and Challenge. Crucially, the questions and their solutions are kept apart. Work through every question in a set on paper before turning to the Solutions section at the very back of the book. Checking as you go, question by question, defeats the purpose. Getting an answer wrong only after genuinely attempting it costs nothing and shows you exactly where to focus, which is the entire point of practising before it matters.

A Quick Reference Formula Sheet, a Glossary, and the Solutions section itself sit at the back of the book, meant for returning to during revision or practice, not for reading straight through. If you ever find yourself relying on the formula sheet without understanding why a formula works, that is a sign to go back to the relevant chapter, not a sign to memorise harder.

Above all, treat mistakes made while working through this book as useful information rather than as evidence of anything about your ability. Every method here was built specifically so that it can be reasoned through from first principles when memory fails under pressure, and that is a skill built through exactly the kind of practice this book is designed to give you.

Before You Begin: Reading the Prescription Safely

Every calculation method in this book starts from information taken off a prescription chart, a medication label, or a pump screen. None of those methods can compensate for information that was misread, misidentified, or unclear in the first place, which is why reading the prescription itself, before any arithmetic begins, deserves its own deliberate step.

Before calculating anything, identify each of the following from the prescription and the medication in front of you: the patient the prescription belongs to, the medicine named, the dose prescribed, the route, the frequency or time, the formulation, the units used, any relevant allergies, whether the prescription is written clearly and unambiguously, and whether the dose looks plausible for this patient and this drug. If anything on that list is unclear, missing, or does not look right, the next step is to clarify it, not to guess, estimate, or proceed anyway.

A note on abbreviations: real prescription charts and drug rounds commonly use shorthand for route and frequency, for example OD for once daily, TDS for three times daily, QDS for four times daily, PRN for when required, and SC for subcutaneous. This book spells these terms out in full throughout, deliberately, so that nothing in the worked examples depends on remembering a shorthand. In practice you will meet the abbreviated forms constantly, and local documentation conventions vary between organisations, so if any abbreviation on a real chart is unfamiliar or ambiguous, checking it before proceeding is exactly the same instinct this section is asking you to build for every other unclear element on a prescription.

This sequence is worth holding in mind as a single flow, from reading through to administration, with the calculation itself sitting in the middle of it rather than at the start:

1. Read the prescription in full

2. Check units and information against the medication available

3. Estimate roughly what the answer should be

4. Calculate precisely

5. Sense-check the calculated answer

6. Check the medicine, concentration, and device against the prescription

7. Administer only if every step above supports it, and escalate if anything does not

Notice that calculation is one step among several, not the whole task. A perfect calculation built on a misread prescription is still an unsafe dose, and a slightly rounded calculation built on careful prescription reading, careful unit checking, and a sound sense-check is very often safer in practice. This book spends most of its pages on the middle of this flow, because that is where the specific mathematical reasoning lives, but every chapter that follows assumes the steps either side of it are being done with equal care.

Reading the Label

MEDICATION CHART EXTRACT	IDENTIFY THESE ELEMENTS
Patient: J. SMITH DOB: 14/03/1958 Drug: Digoxin Dose: 125 micrograms Route: Oral Time: 08:00 Signed: Dr A. Patel	Patient identity Drug name Dose and units Route Time Prescriber signature

Before any calculation, what would you check on a real chart like this?

Every element on the right should be located on the chart before a single number is calculated. Notice how easily "digoxin, 125 micrograms" could be misread as milligrams if scanned quickly, exactly the error this book warns about repeatedly and exactly why writing units in full matters as much on a real chart as it does in a textbook. Practising this identification step deliberately, separately from the arithmetic, is what the flow above is asking of you.

PART I

Build the Foundations

CHAPTER 1

Why Drug Calculations Cause Anxiety (and How This Book Fixes That)

Ask a room full of nursing students which part of the course worries them most, and drug calculations will usually top the list, ahead of anatomy exams, ahead of first clinical placements, sometimes even ahead of finals. This is a strange thing when you think about it. The arithmetic involved in most clinical dose calculations is not advanced. Division, multiplication, working with fractions and decimals, these are skills most people mastered by the end of secondary school. So why does a topic built on relatively simple maths generate this much dread?

The honest answer is that the anxiety rarely comes from the maths itself. It comes from three things layered on top of the maths: the stakes attached to getting it wrong, the way the topic is usually taught, and the pressure of doing the calculation while being watched, timed, or both. Strip those three things away and most people can work through a dose calculation without much trouble. Put them back, and the same calculation suddenly feels much harder than it is.

The Stakes Problem

In almost every other part of the nursing curriculum, a mistake on a practice question costs you nothing beyond a wrong answer and a chance to learn from it. Drug calculations are taught differently from day one, and understandably so, because in real practice a miscalculated dose can cause serious harm. That seriousness is appropriate. Medication errors are a genuine patient safety issue, and calculations sit at the centre of many of them.

The problem is that this seriousness often gets transferred directly into the classroom and the exam hall, without much distinction between practising a skill and performing it under real conditions. Students are told, correctly, that a decimal point error could kill someone, and then handed a worksheet of twenty questions to complete in silence. The result is that every practice question starts to feel like a live clinical decision, which is exactly the kind of pressure that makes ordinary arithmetic mistakes more likely, not less.

This book treats the two situations differently on purpose. While you are learning, the goal is understanding, not performance under pressure. Getting an answer wrong here costs you nothing and tells you exactly where to focus. The habits and checking strategies that keep patients safe are covered in detail later in the book, once the underlying maths is solid. Confidence in the numbers has to come before confidence under pressure. Trying to build both at once is where a lot of the anxiety starts.

The Memorised Formula Trap

Walk into most drug calculation revision sessions and you will see some version of the same formula written on a board: dose required divided by dose available, multiplied by volume or quantity. Students copy it down, apply it to a set of practice questions, and pass the test. Then, weeks or months later, in a placement or an exam, they are handed a slightly unfamiliar question, and the formula stops working, not because it is wrong, but because they never understood why it works in the first place.

A formula memorised without understanding is fragile. It holds up as long as the question looks like the ones you practised on. Change the units, present the information in a different order, add an unfamiliar drug concentration, or simply put the student under time pressure, and the memorised formula falls apart, because there is nothing underneath it to fall back on. This is why so many newly qualified nurses describe passing their calculation exams comfortably and then freezing the first time a real-world question does not match the practice format exactly.

This book takes a different approach. Formulas are not banned, they are genuinely useful shortcuts, but they are introduced only after the reasoning behind them has been built up from first principles. Every method in this book can be re-derived from an understanding of what a dose calculation is actually asking: how much of what you have equals how much of what is needed. Once that idea is solid, formulas become a convenience rather than a crutch, and unfamiliar questions stop being frightening, because you are no longer relying on pattern matching to a memorised template.

It May Not Be a Maths Ability Problem

A significant number of students who struggle with drug calculations describe themselves as "not a maths person." For many people this is worth challenging directly, because it is often untrue, and believing it does real damage. Most people who say this can handle household budgeting, understand discounts and interest rates, follow a recipe that needs scaling up or down, and manage all sorts of everyday numerical reasoning without difficulty. For this group, what is often missing is not the ability to do the maths, but confidence built through the wrong kind of practice, or a bad early experience with the topic that left a lasting impression.

It would be dishonest, though, to suggest this applies to absolutely everyone. Some people genuinely do have a specific numeracy learning need, a diagnosed or undiagnosed processing difficulty such as dyscalculia, a gap left by earlier educational disadvantage, or are working in a language they were not formally schooled in, and any of these can make numerical work harder in a way that is not simply about confidence. If any of this applies to you, that is worth recognising honestly and worth seeking appropriate support for, through your institution's learning support services, rather than being talked out of by blanket reassurance. The distinction that matters practically is the one drawn below: whether the difficulty behaves like a skills gap or like anxiety, because the two call for different responses, and knowing which one you are dealing with, or whether it is some combination of both, is the useful first step, not a label to apply to yourself before checking.

Maths anxiety is a well documented and researched phenomenon, and it behaves differently from a genuine skills gap. A skills gap means the person cannot yet do the calculation. Maths anxiety means the person can do the calculation, under the right conditions, but a switch flips under pressure or under the belief that they are bad at this, and working memory gets used up worrying instead of calculating. The fix for a skills gap is teaching. The fix for anxiety is different: it is repeated, low stakes exposure that rebuilds a track record of success, alongside an honest explanation of what is actually going on mathematically, so the topic stops feeling mysterious.

This book is built around that second kind of fix. Every chapter moves from a plain explanation of the underlying idea, through fully worked examples where every step is shown and justified, to practice questions that let you build a track record of getting things right before speed or pressure enter the picture at all.

How This Book Is Structured

The chapters that follow build in a deliberate order, each one resting on the last. Part One rebuilds core numeracy, fractions, decimals, percentages, ratios, and unit conversion, not as a maths refresher for its own sake, but specifically as it applies to clinical dosing. If any of that feels shaky, do not skip ahead. Almost every calculation error further into the book traces back to a gap in one of these foundations.

Part Two covers tablets, capsules, and oral liquids, the calculations most students meet first and the ones that establish the core reasoning pattern used throughout the rest of the book. Part Three moves into injections and drug concentrations, Part Four into intravenous flow rates, and Part Five into weight based and paediatric dosing, where the stakes and the complexity both increase. Part Six steps back from the arithmetic itself to look at the habits, checking strategies, and mindset that turn calculation competence into calculation safety in real clinical practice.

Each chapter follows the same pattern: a plain language explanation of the idea, several fully worked examples with the reasoning shown at every step, and a set of practice questions with complete solutions. Nothing in this book asks you to trust a formula you do not understand, and nothing skips a step on the assumption that it is obvious. If a step feels obvious to you, that is a good sign, not a reason to feel patronised. It means the foundation is already solid, and the rest of the book will move quickly for you.

A Note on Confidence and Competence

Competence is being able to get the calculation right. Confidence is trusting that you got it right, or knowing how to check when you are not sure. Nursing education has traditionally focused heavily on the first and paid far less attention to the second, which is one reason capable students still feel anxious walking into a drug round. Both matter, because a nurse who is competent but not confident will hesitate, second guess correct work, and take longer than necessary at moments when clarity matters. A nurse who is confident but not competent is a genuine patient safety risk.

This book is written on the basis that patient safety depends on both, and that neither one substitutes for the other. The goal by the end is not just that you can do the calculations, but that you trust yourself to do them, and that the trust is earned rather than assumed.

Key Points

- Drug calculation anxiety usually comes from stakes, teaching methods, and pressure, not from a lack of mathematical ability.
- Memorised formulas fail under unfamiliar conditions because they are not built on understanding.
- Maths anxiety and a genuine skills gap are different problems and need different fixes.

- This book builds understanding first, then introduces formulas as a convenience rather than a starting point.
- Confidence and competence are both necessary for safe practice, and neither one replaces the other.

CHAPTER 2

Core Numeracy Refresher: Fractions, Decimals, Percentages, and Ratios

Every drug calculation you will ever do, no matter how complicated it looks on the surface, is built from four basic numerical ideas: fractions, decimals, percentages, and ratios. This chapter is not a general maths refresher. It focuses specifically on how these four ideas show up in clinical dosing, where they tend to cause trouble, and how to work with them confidently rather than mechanically.

If you already feel solid on this material, read it anyway, briefly. The way these ideas are framed here, in terms of dose and concentration rather than abstract numbers, is the foundation for every method used later in the book. A few minutes now will save confusion in later chapters.

Fractions: What They Actually Represent

A fraction is a comparison between two quantities: how many parts you have, compared to how many parts make up a whole. In clinical dosing, fractions almost always appear in the form of "what you need" over "what you have," written as dose required over dose available. Understanding a fraction this way, as a comparison rather than a piece of abstract notation, is what makes the rest of this book make sense.

The two operations you will use constantly are multiplying fractions and dividing one fraction by another. Multiplying fractions means multiplying the top numbers together and the bottom numbers together. Dividing by a fraction means flipping the second fraction upside down and multiplying instead. This single rule, flip and multiply, underlies far more of drug calculation maths than most students realise.

Worked Example 2.1: Multiplying Fractions

Calculate 3/4 × 2/5.

Step 1: Multiply the top numbers: 3 × 2 = 6.

Step 2: Multiply the bottom numbers: 4 × 5 = 20.

Step 3: The result is 6/20.

Step 4: Simplify by dividing top and bottom by 2: 3/10.

Answer: 3/4 × 2/5 = 3/10

Worked Example 2.2: Dividing by a Fraction

Calculate 1/2 ÷ 3/4.

Step 1: Flip the second fraction: 3/4 becomes 4/3.

Step 2: Change division to multiplication: 1/2 × 4/3.

Step 3: Multiply across: (1 × 4) / (2 × 3) = 4/6.

Step 4: Simplify: 4/6 = 2/3.

Answer: 1/2 ÷ 3/4 = 2/3

Decimals: Precision and Where Errors Hide

Decimals cause more real world medication errors than any other single numerical concept, and almost always for the same reason: a misplaced decimal point. Moving a decimal point one place to the right multiplies a number by ten. Moving it one place to the left divides it by ten. In a clinical context, that single misplaced digit is the difference between a correct dose and a tenfold overdose or underdose, which is why decimal handling deserves more care than any other part of this chapter.

A habit worth building now, and one referenced repeatedly later in this book, is always writing a zero before a decimal point when the number is less than one. Write 0.5, never .5. A stray decimal point in front of an unsupported digit is one of the most common causes of tenfold dosing errors in real clinical practice, because a faint or missed decimal point turns 0.5 into 5. The partner habit, just as important, is to never write an unnecessary trailing zero after a whole number. Write 5 mg, never 5.0 mg, because a poorly printed or handwritten "5.0" can be misread as "50" if the decimal point is missed entirely. The two habits form a single safety rule worth learning as a pair: use a leading zero before a decimal less than one, and avoid an unnecessary trailing zero after a whole number.

Worked Example 2.3: Decimal Multiplication

A vial contains 2.5 mg per mL. How many mg are in 3.2 mL?

Step 1: Multiply 2.5 by 3.2.

Step 2: 2.5 × 3.2 = 2.5 × 3 + 2.5 × 0.2.

Step 3: 2.5 × 3 = 7.5, and 2.5 × 0.2 = 0.5.

Step 4: 7.5 + 0.5 = 8.0.

Answer: 3.2 mL contains 8 mg

Percentages: Concentration in Disguise

A percentage is a fraction out of 100, and in clinical practice it usually describes a concentration, most commonly the strength of a solution. For a solid drug dissolved in a liquid, a 5% solution means 5 grams of a substance dissolved in every 100 mL of fluid. This single fact, that this kind of percentage strength refers to grams per 100 mL, unlocks nearly every percentage-based calculation you will encounter in this book, including a chapter later on injections and reconstitution.

Don't get caught out: percentage strength is not always expressed the same way. What has just been described, grams of solid per 100 mL of liquid, is technically called percentage weight in volume, written % w/v, and it is by far the most common form you will meet in everyday dosing, which is why this book concentrates on it. You may also encounter percentage volume in volume, % v/v, used when both the substance and the diluent are liquids, and percentage weight in weight, % w/w, used for solid or semi-solid preparations such as some creams and ointments. The calculation principle, treating the percentage as a fraction out of 100, is the same in each case, but what that fraction is a fraction of changes. If a percentage strength calculation looks unfamiliar or does not involve a straightforward liquid medicine, check what the percentage is actually describing before assuming it means grams per 100 mL.

To convert a % w/v percentage into a usable amount, treat the percentage sign as an instruction to divide by 100, then apply that fraction to whatever total volume you are working with.

Worked Example 2.4: Percentage Concentration

How many grams of drug are in 250 mL of a 4% solution?

Step 1: A 4% solution contains 4 g per 100 mL.

Step 2: Set up the relationship: 4 g is to 100 mL as x g is to 250 mL.

Step 3: Divide 250 by 100 to find the scaling factor: 2.5.

Step 4: Multiply 4 g by 2.5.

Answer: 250 mL of a 4% solution contains 10 g

Ratios: Comparing Two Quantities Directly

A ratio expresses a relationship between two quantities without necessarily converting it into a fraction or percentage first, and you will meet it most often in drug strengths written as 1 in 1000 or 1:10,000, particularly with medicines like adrenaline. A ratio of 1:1000 means 1 gram of drug in every 1000 mL of solution, or equivalently, 1 mg in every 1 mL, which is worth memorising as a direct conversion because it appears so often in emergency drug calculations.

The safest way to work with ratio strengths is to convert them into a mg per mL figure immediately, before doing anything else with the number. This removes the ratio notation from the rest of the calculation and reduces the chance of a slip later on.

Worked Example 2.5: Ratio Strength Conversion

A drug is supplied as a 1:10,000 solution. How many mg are in 5 mL?

Step 1: 1:10,000 means 1 g in 10,000 mL.

Step 2: Convert 1 g to mg: 1 g = 1000 mg.

Step 3: So the solution contains 1000 mg in 10,000 mL, which simplifies to 0.1 mg per mL.

Step 4: Multiply 0.1 mg by 5 mL.

Answer: 5 mL of a 1:10,000 solution contains 0.5 mg

Rounding in a Clinical Context

Rounding rules in clinical practice are not the same as rounding rules in a maths classroom, because rounding the wrong way at the wrong stage of a calculation can turn a safe dose into an unsafe one. The general clinical principle is to avoid rounding in the middle of a multi-step calculation. Carry full decimal precision through every step, and only round the very last answer, and only to a precision that makes sense for what you are measuring, for example to the nearest whole tablet, the nearest 0.1 mL on a syringe, or the nearest drop per minute on a gravity infusion.

Rounding early and rounding often are two of the most common sources of small but meaningful calculation drift, and this drift compounds in multi-step problems like the IV and paediatric calculations covered later in this book.

Spot the Error

A vial is labelled 1:1000. A student needs to know how many mg are in 3 mL, and calculates it as 1 ÷ 1000 × 3, getting an answer of 0.003 mg.

Before checking the arithmetic, does this figure seem plausible for a 1:1000 strength drug, given what this chapter established about what that ratio actually means?

The arithmetic itself was performed correctly on the wrong starting figure. 1:1000 means 1 g in 1000 mL, which converts to 1 mg per mL, not 1 mg in 1000 mL as the calculation assumed. The correct working is 1 mg per mL × 3 mL, giving 3 mg, a thousand times larger than the flawed answer. This is exactly the kind of error a rough estimate catches immediately: a ratio strength this concentrated should not produce an answer measured in thousandths of a milligram.

Key Points

- Fractions represent a comparison between two quantities, most often dose required over dose available.
- A misplaced decimal point is one of the most common causes of serious medication errors, always write a leading zero before a decimal less than one.
- A percentage concentration usually means grams of substance per 100 mL of solution, specifically for percentage weight in volume, the most common form in everyday dosing.
- A ratio strength such as 1:1000 should be converted into mg per mL before use in any calculation.
- Round only at the final step of a calculation, never in the middle.

CHAPTER 3

Units and Conversions: The Silent Cause of Serious Errors

If decimal point errors are the most common cause of tenfold dosing mistakes, unit conversion errors are close behind, and the two often occur together. A calculation can be arithmetically perfect and still produce a dangerous result if the units feeding into it are inconsistent. This chapter covers the metric system as it is used in clinical practice, the conversions you will use constantly, and the specific points where unit errors tend to creep in unnoticed.

The core message of this chapter is simple to state and easy to forget under pressure: before you calculate anything, make sure every quantity in the problem is in the same unit family, and convert first, calculate second.

The Metric System in Clinical Practice

Nearly all drug calculations in UK clinical practice use the metric system, built around powers of one thousand. Moving from one unit to the next larger or smaller unit means multiplying or dividing by 1000, not by 10 or 100 as some other measurement systems do. This matters because a slip of one zero in either direction represents a thousandfold error, not a small rounding difference.

The units you will use most often, from largest to smallest, are kilograms, grams, milligrams, and micrograms for mass, and litres and millilitres for volume. Each step down divides by 1000: 1 kilogram equals 1000 grams, 1 gram equals 1000 milligrams, and 1 milligram equals 1000 micrograms. The same pattern applies to volume: 1 litre equals 1000 millilitres.

Worked Example 3.1: Converting Milligrams to Micrograms

A prescription states 250 micrograms. The stock is labelled in mg. Convert 250 micrograms to mg.

Step 1: Recall that 1 mg = 1000 micrograms.

Step 2: To convert micrograms to mg, divide by 1000.

Step 3: 250 ÷ 1000 = 0.25.

Answer: 250 micrograms = 0.25 mg

Worked Example 3.2: Converting Grams to Milligrams

A drug chart states a dose of 0.5 g. The available stock is in mg. Convert 0.5 g to mg.

Step 1: Recall that 1 g = 1000 mg.

Step 2: To convert grams to mg, multiply by 1000.

Step 3: 0.5 × 1000 = 500.

Answer: 0.5 g = 500 mg

Why Micrograms Are Never Abbreviated to a Symbol Alone

You will notice that this book, and safe clinical documentation generally, writes "micrograms" in full rather than using the symbol μg. This is a deliberate patient safety convention, not a stylistic choice. The symbol μg can be misread as mg when handwritten quickly or printed in poor quality, and mistaking micrograms for milligrams is a thousandfold error, one of the most dangerous conversion mistakes possible. National medication safety guidance in the UK specifically recommends writing "micrograms" and "nanograms" in full for exactly this reason.

This is a good example of how unit handling is not just a maths issue but a communication and safety issue. Getting the arithmetic right does not help if the units were ambiguous on the chart in the first place.

Converting Body Weight

Weight-based dosing, covered in detail later in this book, depends entirely on an accurate weight in kilograms. Patients and carers sometimes report weight in stones and pounds, particularly with older patients or paediatric weights recorded informally, so converting reliably between these systems and kilograms is a practical necessity, not just an academic exercise.

The conversion to remember is that 1 kilogram is approximately 2.2 pounds. For stones, 1 stone equals 14 pounds, so a weight given in stones and pounds needs to be converted fully to pounds first, then to kilograms.

Worked Example 3.3: Converting Stones and Pounds to Kilograms

A patient weighs 11 stone 4 pounds. Convert this to kilograms.

Step 1: Convert stones to pounds: 11 × 14 = 154 pounds.

Step 2: Add the extra pounds: 154 + 4 = 158 pounds.

Step 3: Convert pounds to kilograms by dividing by 2.2.

Step 4: 158 ÷ 2.2 = 71.8 (to 1 decimal place).

Answer: 11 stone 4 pounds is approximately 71.8 kg

The Golden Rule: Convert First, Calculate Second

The single habit that prevents the majority of unit-related errors is refusing to start a calculation until every number involved is expressed in the same unit. This sounds obvious written down, but it is very easy to skip under time pressure, especially when a dose is prescribed in one unit and the stock available is labelled in another, which happens constantly in real practice.

A simple, practical check before starting any calculation is to write out every given quantity with its unit clearly stated, look at them side by side, and ask whether they match. If a dose is prescribed in micrograms and the vial is labelled in mg, convert one of them before doing anything else. Do not attempt to convert partway through a multiplication or division step, because that is exactly when a conversion error hides inside an otherwise correct-looking calculation.

Spot the Error

A prescription states 500 micrograms. The stock available is labelled 0.25 mg per tablet. A student calculates 500 ÷ 0.25 and gets 2000 tablets.

Before recalculating, what does an answer of 2000 tablets immediately tell you, using nothing more than a general sense of what a normal tablet dose looks like?

It tells you the units were never converted to match before dividing. 0.25 mg is 250 micrograms, not 0.25 micrograms, so dividing 500 by 0.25 compared a quantity in micrograms against a quantity that was still secretly in mg. Converting first, either 500 micrograms to 0.5 mg or 0.25 mg to 250 micrograms, and then dividing two matching units, gives the correct answer of 2 tablets. Keep this example in mind, it resurfaces in Chapter 4 once the tablet calculation method itself has been introduced.

Key Points

- The metric system moves in steps of 1000: kg to g, g to mg, and mg to micrograms.
- A missed or misplaced conversion factor of 1000 is one of the most dangerous errors in clinical dosing.
- Always write "micrograms" and "nanograms" in full, never abbreviate to a symbol that can be misread as mg.
- Convert body weight fully to kilograms before using it in any weight-based calculation.
- Convert every quantity to the same unit before starting a calculation, never mid-calculation.

PART II

Master Everyday Doses

CHAPTER 4

Tablets and Capsules: The Core Method

Tablet and capsule calculations are usually the first drug calculations nursing students meet, and they establish a pattern of reasoning that runs through the entire rest of this book, all the way to IV rates and paediatric weight-based dosing. Get comfortable with the logic in this chapter, and every later chapter will feel like a variation on a theme rather than a new topic.

Every tablet or capsule calculation is answering one question: how many of what I have gives me what has been prescribed. Everything else, including the formula most students memorise, is just a way of writing that question down.

Reading the Label

PRESCRIPTION CHART	STOCK LABEL
Drug: Lisinopril Dose: 15 mg Route: Oral Frequency: once daily	Lisinopril 5 mg tablets 28 tablets

What do you notice before calculating anything?

Two things worth noticing immediately: the prescribed dose and the tablet strength are already in the same unit, mg, so no conversion is needed here, and the numbers suggest a clean, whole-number answer is likely, which is itself a useful early signal. Extracting the right figures from a real chart and a real label, rather than a sentence that hands them to you neatly, is its own small skill, worth practising deliberately alongside the arithmetic itself.

Working this one through: dose required 15 mg, dose available 5 mg, 15 ÷ 5 = 3 tablets.

Building the Method from Understanding

Suppose a prescription asks for 500 mg of a drug, and the tablets available are each 250 mg. Without reaching for any formula, most people can reason this out directly: each tablet supplies 250 mg, so two tablets supply 500 mg. That reasoning, how many times does what I have fit into what I need, is the entire concept behind every tablet calculation.

Written more formally, this becomes dose required divided by dose available. Dose required is the amount prescribed. Dose available is the strength of one tablet or capsule. Dividing the first by the second tells you how many tablets or capsules to give.

It is worth pausing on why division is the correct operation here, rather than simply accepting it as a rule. You are asking how many groups of 250 mg fit inside 500 mg, and finding how many times one quantity fits inside another is exactly what division means. Once this is clear, the formula stops being an arbitrary instruction and becomes a shorthand for reasoning you already understand.

Worked Example 4.1: Basic Tablet Calculation

A patient is prescribed 750 mg of a drug. Tablets are supplied as 250 mg each. How many tablets are needed?

Step 1: Identify dose required: 750 mg.

Step 2: Identify dose available: 250 mg per tablet.

Step 3: Divide dose required by dose available: 750 ÷ 250.

Step 4: 750 ÷ 250 = 3.

Answer: Give 3 tablets

Worked Example 4.2: A Fractional Tablet Result

A patient is prescribed 75 mg of a drug. Tablets are supplied as 50 mg each. How many tablets are needed?

Step 1: Identify dose required: 75 mg.

Step 2: Identify dose available: 50 mg per tablet.

Step 3: Divide: 75 ÷ 50 = 1.5.

Answer: Give 1.5 tablets (1 and a half tablets)

When a Fractional Answer Is and Is Not Acceptable

Worked Example 4.2 produced an answer of one and a half tablets, and whether that is an acceptable instruction depends entirely on the specific formulation in front of you, not on the arithmetic, and not on a simple rule of thumb. It is tempting to reach for a general rule, such as scored tablets can be split and everything else cannot, but whether a tablet can be divided, or a capsule opened, is preparation-specific, and general rules of this kind can be wrong in both directions. Some modified release capsules, for example, are designed to be opened as long as their internal granules are not crushed or chewed, while some scored tablets should still not be split due to how the drug is distributed within them. UK specialist pharmacy guidance is explicit that this must be checked against the product's own literature or a medicines information source, not assumed from the tablet's appearance.

The safe practice is therefore: never assume that a tablet can be divided, crushed, or dispersed, or that a capsule can be opened, based on its appearance or on a general rule. Check the product information, a medicines reference such as the current edition of the relevant formulary, or pharmacy guidance, every time this situation arises. This is a case where the maths and the clinical decision are genuinely separate steps. The calculation tells you the number that satisfies the prescribed dose. Whether that number is deliverable safely with the specific formulation in front of you is a professional judgement that sits on top of the arithmetic, not a replacement for it. If a calculation produces a fractional result and there is any doubt about whether the formulation can be safely divided, the appropriate response is to check the product information or contact pharmacy, not to guess.

Multiple Strengths and Combination Dosing

Sometimes a single tablet strength cannot deliver the prescribed dose in a sensible number of tablets, and more than one strength is available on the ward. The same dose required over dose available logic still applies, it is simply applied to select the most practical combination, generally preferring the fewest number of tablets and whole tablets over split ones wherever possible.

Worked Example 4.3: Choosing Between Available Strengths

A patient is prescribed 300 mg of a drug. Both 100 mg and 150 mg tablets are available. What is the most practical combination?

Step 1: Check 150 mg tablets first: 300 ÷ 150 = 2.

Step 2: Two 150 mg tablets give exactly 300 mg with no splitting required.

Step 3: Compare with 100 mg tablets: 300 ÷ 100 = 3, which would need three tablets instead of two.

Step 4: Two whole tablets is the more practical choice.

Answer: Give two 150 mg tablets

A Quick Sense-Check Habit

Before finalising any tablet calculation, it is worth asking whether the answer feels plausible. A patient being given fifteen tablets for a routine oral dose, or a fraction of a tablet for a drug that is not available in a smaller strength, should immediately raise a flag. In the vast majority of real prescribing, sensible tablet counts fall within a small range, typically one to four tablets per dose. An answer well outside that range is far more likely to indicate a unit error, a misread prescription, or a decimal point slip than an unusual clinical situation, and is worth rechecking before proceeding.

A Framework: Before You Calculate

From here on, it is worth running through a short mental checklist before touching a calculator on any clinical dosing question, not just tablets. It takes seconds once it becomes a habit, and it catches a surprising number of errors before they happen, because it forces the reasoning that a rushed calculation skips past.

Before you calculate: what am I actually being asked to find. What unit should my answer have. Are all my quantities currently in the same unit, or does something need converting first. Roughly what answer should I expect. Only once those four questions have an answer, calculate precisely. Then, after calculating: does my answer make clinical sense. This last question is the sense-check habit already introduced above, and the four questions before it are simply that same habit, moved to the start of the process instead of the end, where it can prevent an error rather than only catch one after the fact.

Spot the Error

A prescription asks for 500 micrograms. The stock available is labelled 0.25 mg per tablet. A student works the calculation as 500 ÷ 0.25 and gets 2000 tablets. This is the same scenario flagged at the end of Chapter 3, worth revisiting now that the tablet method itself is in view.

Stop before recalculating. What tells you immediately that 2000 tablets cannot be right, without checking a single step of the arithmetic?

The plausibility check from this chapter is the giveaway: a typical tablet dose falls somewhere between one and four tablets. Two thousand is so far outside that range that the answer is wrong before any arithmetic is reviewed at all. As Chapter 3 established, the actual error is a missed unit conversion: 0.25 mg is 250 micrograms, not 0.25 micrograms, so the two figures were never in the same unit to begin with. Converting first, 500 micrograms ÷ 250 micrograms, gives the correct answer of 2 tablets. Notice that this chapter and the last one catch the same error two different ways, one by checking the units before dividing, one by checking the plausibility of the answer afterwards. Using both together is stronger than relying on either alone.

Key Points

- The tablet calculation method is dose required divided by dose available.
- This division answers the question of how many times the available strength fits into the prescribed dose.
- Never assume a tablet can be split or a capsule opened. Check the product information or pharmacy guidance every time.
- A fractional result where there is any doubt about splitting means checking the product information, not rounding or guessing.
- Before calculating, check what you're finding, what unit it should be in, whether your quantities already match, and roughly what to expect. An unusually large or small answer is a signal to recheck before administering.

CHAPTER 5

Liquid Medications and Oral Suspensions

Liquid medications use exactly the same reasoning as tablets and capsules, with one addition: the answer is a volume rather than a count of solid units. Where a tablet calculation asks how many discrete units to give, a liquid calculation asks how many millilitres contain the prescribed dose. The underlying logic, dose required compared against dose available, does not change at all.

Reading the Label

PRESCRIPTION CHART	STOCK LABEL
Drug: Amoxicillin Dose: 375 mg Route: Oral Frequency: three times daily	Amoxicillin Susp. 125 mg in 5 mL SHAKE WELL

What do you notice before calculating anything?

The units already match, both in mg, so this is purely a matter of applying the liquid formula rather than converting anything first. Notice too the printed instruction to shake the bottle, which Chapter 5 explains is not a formality, it directly affects whether the concentration you draw up matches the concentration on the label. Working this through: dose required 375 mg, dose available 125 mg, volume 5 mL. 375 ÷ 125 = 3, then 3 × 5 mL = 15 mL.

Extending the Method to Volume

A liquid medication is always labelled with a concentration, expressed as an amount of drug per a stated volume, for example 250 mg in 5 mL. This is the dose available, but unlike a tablet, it is not a single indivisible unit, it is a strength attached to a volume that can be measured in any amount. The calculation therefore has three quantities rather than two: the dose required, the dose available, and the volume that the dose available occupies.

The method is: divide the dose required by the dose available, then multiply the result by the volume the dose available is dissolved in. Written as a formula, this is dose required over dose available, multiplied by volume. This is the same formula seen in tablet calculations, with an extra multiplication step to account for the fact that the available strength is spread across a specific volume rather than sitting in one physical unit.

Worked Example 5.1: Basic Liquid Calculation

A patient is prescribed 500 mg of a drug. It is available as a suspension of 250 mg in 5 mL. How many mL should be given?

Step 1: Identify dose required: 500 mg.

Step 2: Identify dose available: 250 mg.

Step 3: Identify the volume the dose available occupies: 5 mL.

Step 4: Divide dose required by dose available: 500 ÷ 250 = 2.

Step 5: Multiply by the volume: 2 × 5 mL = 10 mL.

Answer: Give 10 mL

Worked Example 5.2: A Less Convenient Concentration

A patient is prescribed 125 mg of a drug, available as 250 mg in 10 mL. How many mL should be given?

Step 1: Dose required: 125 mg. Dose available: 250 mg. Volume: 10 mL.

Step 2: Divide: 125 ÷ 250 = 0.5.

Step 3: Multiply by volume: 0.5 × 10 mL = 5 mL.

Answer: Give 5 mL

Suspensions Need Shaking, and Why That Matters Mathematically

A suspension is a liquid medication in which the drug particles are dispersed through the liquid rather than fully dissolved, and if it is left standing, those particles settle toward the bottom of the container. This is not just a pharmacy instruction to be followed out of habit, it directly affects the accuracy of the calculation you have just done. A calculation assumes the concentration stated on the label, for example 250 mg in 5 mL, is uniform throughout the bottle. If the suspension has not been shaken thoroughly, the liquid drawn from the top of the bottle may contain significantly less drug than the label states, and the liquid from the bottom may contain more, regardless of how precisely the calculation itself was performed.

This is a useful example of a wider point that recurs throughout this book. A perfectly correct calculation still depends on the real-world conditions matching the assumptions the calculation was based on. Always shake a suspension thoroughly immediately before measuring a dose.

Measuring Accurately: Oral Syringes and Spoons

Household spoons are not a reliable measuring device and should never be used for medication dosing, because their volume varies considerably between different spoons, sometimes by as much as double. Oral doses should always be measured using an oral syringe or a manufacturer-supplied measuring device with clear graduations. Oral syringes are generally graduated in increments of 0.1 mL to 1 mL depending on their size, and doses should be rounded to the nearest measurable increment on the device actually being used, not to an arbitrary number of decimal places.

This connects directly back to the rounding principle from Chapter 2. The calculation itself should be carried out with full precision, and only the final answer is rounded, and only to a precision the measuring device can actually achieve. A calculated dose of 4.37 mL, for example, might be rounded to 4.4 mL on a syringe graduated in 0.1 mL increments, but there is no value in calculating to two decimal places if the equipment cannot measure that precisely.

Reading the Label

PRESCRIPTION CHART	ORAL SYRINGE
Drug: Paracetamol Dose: 180 mg Route: Oral Frequency: four times daily, when required	120 mg in 5 mL Size: 10 mL Graduations: 0.1 mL

What do you notice before calculating anything?

Notice the syringe's capacity as well as its graduations. A device with fine graduations is only useful if it can actually hold the calculated volume in one measurement. Working through the figures: dose required 180 mg, dose available 120 mg, volume 5 mL. 180 ÷ 120 = 1.5, × 5 mL = 7.5 mL, a volume that needs at least a 10 mL oral syringe, not the smaller 5 mL size a quicker glance might reach for.

Worked Example 5.3: Rounding to a Measurable Increment

A calculation produces a required dose of 6.23 mL, to be measured using an oral syringe graduated in 0.1 mL increments. What volume should actually be drawn up?

Step 1: The syringe can only measure in steps of 0.1 mL.

Step 2: 6.23 mL falls between the 6.2 mL and 6.3 mL markings.

Step 3: 6.23 is closer to 6.2 than to 6.3.

Step 4: Round to the nearest available increment.

Answer: Draw up 6.2 mL

Let the Units Check Your Maths

There is a simple visual habit worth adding to the liquid calculation method covered in this chapter, and it works by making the units themselves confirm that a calculation is set up correctly, before you even reach a final number. Write the calculation out with every unit attached to its figure, not just the numbers, and look at which units would cancel if you multiplied straight across.

For the calculation in Worked Example 5.1, 500 mg over 250 mg, multiplied by 5 mL, the mg on the top and the mg on the bottom cancel each other out, leaving only mL, which is exactly the unit the answer should be in. If a calculation is set up backwards, the units will not cancel to leave the unit you expect, and that mismatch is visible before you finish the arithmetic, not just after. Some textbooks call this dimensional analysis, but there is nothing complicated about it, it is simply letting the units confirm the answer belongs in mL, or mg, or whatever unit the question is actually asking for. Think of it as a built-in version of the sense-check habit from Chapter 4, applied directly to the structure of the calculation rather than to the size of the final number.

Key Points

- Liquid dose calculations use dose required over dose available, multiplied by the volume the available strength occupies.
- Suspensions must be shaken thoroughly before measuring, or the concentration drawn up will not match the label.
- Never use a household spoon to measure a medical dose, always use an oral syringe or supplied measuring device.
- Round the final answer only, and only to the smallest increment the measuring device can actually deliver.
- Writing out units alongside every figure and checking that they cancel to leave the expected unit is a quick way to confirm a calculation is set up correctly.

CHAPTER 6

Practice Set 1: Tablets, Capsules, and Liquid Medications

The fourteen questions in this chapter draw on everything covered so far: core numeracy, unit conversion, tablet and capsule calculations, and liquid medication calculations. They are deliberately mixed rather than grouped by type, because real clinical practice does not sort itself into neat categories, and part of building genuine confidence is being able to recognise which method a question needs without being told in advance.

Work through every question below yourself, on paper, before turning to the Solutions section at the back of the book. Resist the urge to check as you go, question by question, since that is exactly the habit that stops genuine independent practice from happening. When you do check, if you get an answer wrong, do not just note the correct figure and move on. Find the specific step where your reasoning diverged from the solution shown, because that is the exact gap worth closing before moving into the next part of the book.

Question 1 · Foundation

A patient is prescribed 1 g of a drug. Tablets are available in 500 mg strength. How many tablets should be given?

Question 2 · Foundation

A prescription states 62.5 micrograms. Tablets are available in 0.125 mg strength. How many tablets should be given?

Question 3 · Foundation

A patient is prescribed 375 mg of a drug, available as a suspension of 125 mg in 5 mL. How many mL should be given?

Question 4 · Clinical Application

A patient is prescribed 180 mg of a drug, available as 300 mg in 10 mL. How many mL should be given, rounded to a syringe graduated in 0.1 mL increments?

Question 5 · Clinical Application

How many grams of drug are contained in 40 mL of a 10% solution?

Question 6 · Clinical Application

A drug is supplied as a 1:1000 solution. How many mg are contained in 2 mL?

Question 7 · Challenge

A patient is prescribed 450 mg of a drug. Tablets are available in both 150 mg and 225 mg strengths. What is the most practical combination?

Question 8 · Challenge

A patient is prescribed 0.6 g of a drug, available as a suspension of 240 mg in 5 mL. How many mL should be given?

Question 9 · Foundation

A patient is prescribed 250 mg of a drug. Tablets are available in 125 mg strength. How many tablets should be given?

Question 10 · Foundation

Convert 0.75 g to mg.

Question 11 · Clinical Application

A patient is prescribed 90 mg of a drug, available as a suspension of 60 mg in 5 mL. How many mL should be given?

Question 12 · Clinical Application

A patient is prescribed 800 micrograms of a drug. Tablets are available in 0.4 mg strength. How many tablets should be given?

Question 13 · Challenge

A patient is prescribed 0.9 g of a drug per day, available as a suspension of 300 mg in 10 mL, to be given in three divided doses. How many mL should be given per dose?

Question 14 · Challenge

A calculation for a patient prescribed 600 mg, using a stock strength of 200 mg per tablet, is worked as 200 ÷ 600, giving 0.33. What does this suggest, and what is the correct answer?

How Did You Do?

If you worked through all fourteen questions correctly, on your own, without checking the solution until you had committed to an answer, that is a genuine sign that the reasoning from the last four chapters has taken hold. If you got some wrong, look specifically at whether the error was a unit conversion missed at the start, a decimal or fraction slip in the middle, or a misjudgement about whether a fractional result was clinically appropriate. Each of those is a different kind of gap, and knowing which one it was tells you exactly which earlier chapter is worth another look before moving on to injections in Part Three.

PART III

Injections and High-Risk Medicines

CHAPTER 7

Calculating Injection Volumes

Injectable medications introduce two new practical considerations on top of the maths already covered: choosing the right syringe to measure the volume accurately, and, for some drugs, reconstituting a powder into a solution before any dose can be drawn up at all. The underlying calculation is the same dose required over dose available method used for oral liquids. What changes is the precision required and the extra step some medications need before that formula can even be applied.

Reading the Label

PRESCRIPTION CHART	AMPOULE LABEL
Drug: Morphine Sulfate Dose: 7.5 mg Route: subcutaneous Frequency: when required, 4 hourly	Morphine Sulfate 10 mg in 1 mL For subcutaneous or intramuscular use

What do you notice before calculating anything?

This is an opioid, a high-risk drug by the definition covered later in Chapter 12, which is itself worth registering before touching the calculation, since it signals that extra checking may be required by local policy regardless of how straightforward the arithmetic turns out to be. The units match, both mg, so no conversion is needed. Working it through: dose required 7.5 mg, dose available 10 mg, volume 1 mL. $7.5 \div 10 = 0.75$, $\times$ 1 mL = 0.75 mL, a volume small enough that a 1 mL syringe graduated in 0.01 mL increments is the appropriate choice, not a larger, coarser one.

The Same Method, Higher Stakes

An injection calculation asks exactly the same question as an oral liquid calculation: how many mL contain the prescribed dose, given the concentration of the solution available. The formula is unchanged, dose required divided by dose available, multiplied by the volume the available strength occupies. What changes with injections is the margin for error. Injectable doses often involve smaller volumes, more potent drugs, and routes that bypass the body's natural absorption safeguards, so a calculation error reaches the bloodstream faster and with less opportunity to intervene than an oral dosing error.

Worked Example 7.1: Basic Injection Volume

A patient is prescribed 40 mg of a drug by intramuscular injection. It is supplied as 80 mg in 2 mL. How many mL should be drawn up?

Step 1: Dose required: 40 mg. Dose available: 80 mg. Volume: 2 mL.

Step 2: Divide: 40 ÷ 80 = 0.5.

Step 3: Multiply by volume: 0.5 × 2 mL = 1 mL.

Answer: Draw up 1 mL

Choosing the Right Syringe

Syringes are manufactured in a range of sizes, commonly 1 mL, 2 mL, 5 mL, 10 mL and larger, and each size has different graduation increments printed along the barrel. A 1 mL syringe is typically marked in increments of 0.01 mL, making it the right choice for small, precise volumes such as paediatric doses or potent drugs given in fractions of a millilitre. A 2 mL or 5 mL syringe is usually marked in increments of 0.1 mL, and larger syringes still may only be marked in whole millilitres.

The general safety principle is to choose the smallest syringe that will comfortably hold the required volume, because a smaller syringe gives finer graduations and therefore a more accurate measurement. Drawing up 0.4 mL in a 5 mL syringe marked only in 0.2 mL increments is far less precise than drawing up the same volume in a 1 mL syringe marked in 0.01 mL increments, even though the calculation producing that 0.4 mL figure was identical in both cases.

Reading the Label

PRESCRIPTION CHART	1 mL SYRINGE SCALE
Drug: Glycopyrronium Dose: 120 micrograms Route: subcutaneous Frequency: when required	0.0 . 0.1 . 0.2 . 0.3 0.4 . 0.5 . 0.6 . 0.7 0.8 . 0.9 . 1.0 (0.01 mL graduations)

What do you notice before calculating anything?

The stock, mentioned on the drug's ampoule as 200 micrograms in 1 mL, and the syringe pictured here are both graduated finely enough to matter for this dose. Working it through: dose required 120 micrograms, dose available 200 micrograms, volume 1 mL. 120 ÷ 200 = 0.6, × 1 mL = 0.6 mL, a figure that lands precisely on a marked graduation on this scale rather than between two markings, which is worth noticing, since not every calculated volume will land so neatly.

Worked Example 7.2: Selecting an Appropriate Syringe

A calculation produces a required volume of 0.35 mL. Which syringe size is most appropriate: 1 mL, 2 mL, or 5 mL?

Step 1: 0.35 mL is a small volume relative to the capacity of a 2 mL or 5 mL syringe.

Step 2: A 1 mL syringe, typically graduated in 0.01 mL increments, can measure 0.35 mL precisely.

Step 3: A 2 mL or 5 mL syringe, graduated in larger increments, would force rounding to a less accurate figure.

Answer: Use a 1 mL syringe

Reconstitution: Turning a Powder into a Solution

Some injectable drugs are unstable in liquid form and are supplied as a dry powder, to be dissolved in a diluent, usually water for injection or normal saline, immediately before use. This process is called reconstitution, and it must happen before any dose calculation can be applied, because a powder alone has no meaningful concentration in mg per mL until it has been dissolved in a specific, known volume.

The manufacturer's instructions, printed on the packaging or the accompanying literature, state exactly how much diluent to add to produce a specific final concentration. This instruction must always be followed precisely and never estimated, because adding more or less diluent than specified changes the final concentration, which then changes every calculation that follows from it. Once reconstituted according to the instructions, the resulting solution is treated exactly like any other liquid medication, with a known concentration to which the standard dose required over dose available method applies directly.

Reading the Label

PRESCRIPTION CHART	VIAL LABEL
Drug: Cefuroxime Dose: 500 mg Route: IV Frequency: three times daily	Cefuroxime 750 mg Powder for Injection Reconstitute with 6 mL WFI per product literature

What do you notice before calculating anything, and how is this different from the ampoule earlier in this chapter?

Unlike the ampoule earlier in this chapter, which already contained a ready-to-use solution, this vial contains a dry powder with no meaningful concentration at all until it has been reconstituted exactly as instructed, 6 mL of water for injection added to give 750 mg in 6 mL. Only once that step is complete does the standard method apply: dose required 500 mg, dose available 750 mg, volume 6 mL. 500 ÷ 750 = 0.67, × 6 mL = 4 mL.

Worked Example 7.3: Calculating a Dose After Reconstitution

A powder for injection is reconstituted according to the manufacturer's instructions to produce a solution of 500 mg in 4 mL. A patient is prescribed 250 mg. How many mL should be given?

Step 1: Confirm reconstitution has been carried out exactly as per the manufacturer's instructions, producing 500 mg in 4 mL.

Step 2: Dose required: 250 mg. Dose available: 500 mg. Volume: 4 mL.

Step 3: Divide: 250 ÷ 500 = 0.5.

Step 4: Multiply by volume: 0.5 × 4 mL = 2 mL.

Answer: Give 2 mL

A Note on Displacement Volume

One detail worth being aware of, though full working is beyond the scope of this chapter, is that some powders take up measurable space once dissolved, known as displacement volume. If a manufacturer's instructions specify adding 3.5 mL of diluent to achieve a particular concentration, this figure has already accounted for the powder's displacement volume, so the instructions should be followed exactly as written rather than adjusted. Displacement volume only becomes something to calculate manually in specific situations, such as certain paediatric or highly concentrated preparations, and where this applies, local policy and the manufacturer's literature will specify the calculation required. When in doubt, checking with pharmacy is always the safe default.

Key Points

- Injection volume calculations use the same dose required over dose available formula as oral liquids.

- Choose the smallest syringe that comfortably holds the required volume, for the finest available graduation.
- A powder must be reconstituted exactly per the manufacturer's instructions before any dose calculation applies.
- Never estimate a diluent volume during reconstitution, incorrect diluent volume changes the resulting concentration.
- Displacement volume is usually already accounted for in manufacturer instructions, check with pharmacy if unsure.

CHAPTER 8

Understanding Drug Concentrations: Units, Insulin, and Heparin

Every concentration covered so far in this book, mg per mL, percentage solutions, ratio strengths, has ultimately been a measure of mass, an amount of substance that can be weighed. This chapter covers a different kind of measurement entirely: the unit, used for a small number of high-risk drugs including insulin and heparin, where the standard mass-based approach does not apply and treating it as if it did is a serious and well-documented source of harm.

What a Unit Actually Measures

A unit is a measure of biological activity or potency, not a measure of mass. It exists because certain substances, insulin among them, cannot be dosed reliably by weight alone, since the biological effect of a given mass can vary between manufacturing batches or preparation methods. Instead, the drug is standardised so that one unit always produces a consistent, defined biological effect, regardless of how many milligrams of the substance that unit happens to correspond to.

The practical consequence is that units and milligrams are not interchangeable, and there is no universal conversion factor between them that applies across different drugs. A unit of insulin and a unit of heparin measure completely different things and cannot be compared to each other, or converted to milligrams, using any formula in this book or elsewhere. When a drug is prescribed and supplied in units, the entire calculation, from prescription to administration, stays in units throughout. This is the single most important idea in this chapter, and one worth returning to if any part of this section feels unclear.

Insulin: Units, Concentrations, and Device Safety

Insulin has traditionally been supplied in the UK at a standardised concentration of 100 units per mL, commonly written as U-100, and this is still by far the most common strength in general use. It is a mistake, however, to assume every insulin preparation is U-100. Higher-strength insulin preparations, including 200 units per mL and 300 units per mL products, are in routine clinical use, and UK medicines safety guidance specifically warns about the medication-error risk these higher strengths carry, precisely because a nurse who assumes U-100 by habit can seriously under- or overestimate a dose drawn from a different strength device.

The safe practice this creates is straightforward to state and important to follow without exception: always check the specific insulin product name, its concentration, and the device it is supplied in, every time, rather than assuming a familiar concentration. Always use the administration device appropriate to the specific insulin product. Where insulin is supplied in a pre-filled pen, use the pen as directed, dialling the prescribed number of units directly, and never withdraw insulin from a pen into a separate syringe. Using a standard mL syringe to draw up insulin, reading the barrel markings as if they represented units, is a well documented and dangerous error regardless of the concentration involved, because a standard syringe is graduated in mL, not units, and the number of units in each mL depends entirely on which strength of insulin is in front of you.

Never independently convert or adjust an insulin pen dose because the concentration differs from what you expected. Pens are designed to dial and deliver a dose in units regardless of the concentration inside them, and a mismatch between the prescribed insulin and the device available should be resolved by checking the prescription and product against local insulin policy, not by working out a manual conversion at the bedside. Because insulin syringes and pens are calibrated directly in units, most routine insulin administration does not require the dose required over dose available formula at all. The prescribed number of units is dialled or drawn up directly on a device that reads in units. The calculation becomes necessary primarily when insulin is being prepared for an infusion, where a specific concentration in units per mL needs to be established in a larger volume of fluid, and even then, local insulin infusion policy and manufacturer guidance take precedence over any general method shown here.

Dose-step check: the dose counter on an insulin pen displays the dose in units, irrespective of insulin strength, as established above. However, different pen devices may deliver doses in different dose-step increments, current UK guidance highlights that older devices typically step in whole units, some newer high-strength pens step in 2-unit increments, and some paediatric formulations step in as little as 0.5 units. Always confirm that the prescribed dose is achievable on the specific pen device in front of you. If it is not, for example a prescribed odd number of units on a device that only steps in twos, do not improvise, round, or attempt a manual conversion to a different device. Check the product information and seek pharmacy or prescriber advice.

Reading the Label

PRESCRIPTION CHART	PEN DISPLAY
Drug: Insulin Glargine Dose: 24 units Route: subcutaneous Frequency: once daily, evening	300 units/mL DIAL WINDOW: 24 units

What do you notice before calculating anything?

There is nothing to calculate here at all, and recognising that is the actual skill being tested. The pen dials directly in units, so the 300 units per mL concentration printed on it does not change what number to dial, 24. The concentration would only become relevant if this insulin were ever withdrawn from the pen into a separate syringe, which safe practice avoids for pen-supplied insulin precisely for this reason. The correct action is simply to dial 24 and administer, having confirmed the product and pen are correct for this patient.

Worked Example 8.1: Preparing an Insulin Infusion

An insulin infusion is to be prepared at a concentration of 1 unit per mL, using 50 units of insulin made up to a total volume with sodium chloride 0.9%. What total volume should the insulin be made up to?

Step 1: The target concentration is 1 unit per mL.

Step 2: Total units available: 50 units.

Step 3: To achieve 1 unit per mL, the total volume must equal the total number of units.

Step 4: 50 units at 1 unit per mL requires a total volume of 50 mL.

Answer: Make up to a total volume of 50 mL

Heparin: Units in a Larger Volume

Heparin is supplied in a range of concentrations expressed in units per mL, and unlike insulin, there is no single standardised strength, which makes checking the specific concentration on the vial or ampoule before every calculation essential. Heparin doses can be given as a single bolus injection or as a continuous infusion, and infusion doses are often prescribed in units per hour, requiring a further step to convert an hourly dose into a pump rate in mL per hour, a calculation covered in detail in the next part of this book alongside other IV rate calculations.

For a straightforward bolus dose, the calculation follows the same logical structure used throughout this book, substituting units for mg, dose required over dose available, multiplied by volume, as long as the required dose and the available concentration are both expressed in units.

Worked Example 8.2: Heparin Bolus Dose

A patient is prescribed a heparin bolus of 4000 units. It is supplied as 5000 units in 5 mL. How many mL should be given?

Step 1: Dose required: 4000 units. Dose available: 5000 units. Volume: 5 mL.

Step 2: Divide: 4000 ÷ 5000 = 0.8.

Step 3: Multiply by volume: 0.8 × 5 mL = 4 mL.

Answer: Give 4 mL

Never Abbreviate the Word "Units"

National medication safety guidance is explicit that the word "units" must always be written in full and never abbreviated to "U" or "IU." This is not a stylistic preference, it is a documented patient safety measure. A handwritten or poorly printed "U" can be misread as a zero, so a dose of 4U can be misread as 40, a tenfold error, or an "IU" can be misread as "IV," changing the intended route entirely. These are not hypothetical risks, they are recurring, recognised causes of serious medication incidents involving insulin in particular, and they are entirely preventable simply by writing the word out in full every time.

Key Points

- A unit measures biological activity, not mass, and units cannot be converted to milligrams.
- Insulin is commonly U-100, but higher-strength preparations exist. Always check the specific product and concentration, and always measure using the device it is supplied in, never a standard mL syringe.
- Heparin concentrations vary between preparations, always check the specific strength on the vial before calculating.
- The dose required over dose available method still applies to unit-based drugs, as long as every quantity is expressed consistently in units.
- Always write "units" in full. Never abbreviate to U or IU, both are recognised causes of serious dosing errors.

CHAPTER 9

Practice Set 2: Injections, Reconstitution, and Unit-Based Dosing

This set covers Part Three in full: injection volumes, syringe selection, reconstitution, and unit-based drugs including insulin and heparin. Fourteen questions this time, one of which asks you to identify an error rather than calculate an answer, because recognising an unsafe calculation is just as important a skill as producing a correct one. Work through all fourteen questions before turning to the Solutions section at the back of the book.

Question 1 · Foundation

A patient is prescribed 15 mg of a drug by subcutaneous injection. It is supplied as 30 mg in 3 mL. How many mL should be given?

Question 2 · Foundation

A calculation produces a required volume of 0.22 mL. Which syringe is most appropriate: a 1 mL syringe graduated in 0.01 mL, or a 2 mL syringe graduated in 0.1 mL?

Question 3 · Foundation

A powder for injection is reconstituted per the manufacturer's instructions to give a solution of 1 g in 10 mL. A patient is prescribed 400 mg. How many mL should be given?

Question 4 · Clinical Application

A patient is prescribed a heparin bolus of 7500 units. It is supplied as 25,000 units in 5 mL. How many mL should be given?

Question 5 · Clinical Application

An insulin infusion is to be prepared at 1 unit per mL using 40 units of insulin made up with sodium chloride 0.9%. What total volume should the insulin be made up to?

Question 6 · Clinical Application

A patient is prescribed 300 micrograms of a drug by injection. It is supplied as 0.5 mg in 1 mL. How many mL should be given?

Question 7 · Challenge

A patient is prescribed 600 mg of a drug by injection. Two vial strengths are available: 300 mg in 2 mL, and 600 mg in 4 mL. Which is the more practical choice, and what volume is drawn up?

Question 8 · Challenge: Spot the Error

A nurse is asked to draw up 12 units of insulin. Finding no insulin syringe available, they draw up 0.12 mL of U-100 insulin using a standard 1 mL syringe, reasoning that the markings can be read directly as units. Is this calculation and approach safe?

Question 9 · Foundation

A patient is prescribed 20 mg of a drug by injection, supplied as 40 mg in 2 mL. How many mL should be drawn up?

Question 10 · Foundation

A drug is supplied as a 1:10,000 solution. How many mg are in 10 mL?

Question 11 · Clinical Application

A patient is prescribed a heparin bolus of 5000 units, supplied as 25,000 units in 5 mL. How many mL should be given?

Question 12 · Clinical Application

A powder for injection is reconstituted per the manufacturer's instructions to give 250 mg in 2 mL. A patient is prescribed 150 mg. How many mL should be given?

Question 13 · Challenge

A calculation produces a required volume of 0.18 mL. Two syringes are available: a 1 mL syringe graduated in 0.01 mL, and a 2 mL syringe graduated in 0.1 mL. Which should be used, and why does it matter here specifically?

Question 14 · Challenge

A nurse checks a heparin vial and finds it labelled 1000 units per mL, having expected the 5000 units per mL strength used on the same ward yesterday. What should the nurse do?

How Did You Do?

Question 8 was included deliberately to make a point that runs through this entire book: correct arithmetic is necessary but is not, by itself, the same thing as a safe clinical decision. If you flagged the syringe choice as the problem before reading the solution, that is exactly the kind of clinical judgement this book is trying to build alongside the calculation skills themselves. Part Four moves into intravenous flow rates, where this same principle, correct maths plus correct clinical judgement, becomes even more important.

PART IV

Intravenous Calculations

CHAPTER 10

Calculating IV Flow Rates

Intravenous fluids and medications are given at a controlled rate over time, and calculating that rate correctly is one of the highest-stakes calculations in this book, because an IV rate that is too fast can cause fluid overload or a dangerously rapid drug delivery, and a rate that is too slow can mean a patient does not receive treatment on the timescale intended. This chapter covers the two main ways an IV rate is delivered and calculated: through an electronic infusion pump, set in millilitres per hour, and through a gravity-fed giving set, counted in drops per minute.

Reading the Label

PRESCRIPTION CHART	PUMP SCREEN
Fluid: Sod. Chloride 0.9% Volume: 1000 mL Duration: 8 hours Route: IV	VOLUME: 1000 mL TIME: --- hrs RATE: --- mL/hr PRESS SET

What do you notice before calculating anything?

The pump screen is asking for a rate, not just displaying one, which is exactly the figure this calculation needs to produce before the pump can actually be programmed. The volume and duration on the chart are already what the formula needs, with no unit conversion required here. Working it through: 1000 mL ÷ 8 hours = 125 mL per hour, the figure that belongs in the pump's RATE field.

Millilitres per Hour: The Pump Calculation

An infusion pump is programmed with a rate in mL per hour, and the calculation behind that rate is a direct application of an idea you already know well: how much divided by how long. If a certain volume of fluid needs to be given over a certain number of hours, the rate in mL per hour is simply the total volume divided by the total time in hours.

This is the same underlying logic as every calculation so far in this book, comparing one quantity against another, just applied to volume and time rather than dose and concentration.

Worked Example 10.1: Basic mL per Hour Calculation

A patient is prescribed 1 litre of sodium chloride 0.9% to be given over 8 hours via an infusion pump. What rate, in mL per hour, should the pump be set to?

Step 1: Convert the volume to mL: 1 litre = 1000 mL.

Step 2: Divide the total volume by the total time: 1000 ÷ 8.

Step 3: 1000 ÷ 8 = 125.

Answer: Set the pump to 125 mL per hour

Worked Example 10.2: Working Backwards from Rate to Duration

A 500 mL bag is being infused at 100 mL per hour. How long will the infusion take to complete?

Step 1: This question reverses the previous logic: time equals volume divided by rate.

Step 2: Divide the total volume by the rate: 500 ÷ 100.

Step 3: 500 ÷ 100 = 5.

Answer: The infusion will take 5 hours

Drops per Minute: The Gravity Infusion Calculation

Not every clinical area uses electronic pumps for every infusion, and gravity-fed giving sets, controlled by adjusting a roller clamp and counting drops falling in a chamber, are still used, particularly in some community, hospice, and lower-acuity settings. Because a drop is not a standard unit of volume, the calculation depends on a specific piece of information printed on the giving set packaging:

the drop factor, which states how many drops of that particular set equal 1 mL.

As a general guide, solution giving sets are commonly around 20 drops per mL, blood and blood product giving sets are commonly around 15 drops per mL, reflecting the higher viscosity of blood, and paediatric or burette giving sets, sometimes called microdrop sets, are commonly around 60 drops per mL, allowing smaller volumes to be delivered with usable accuracy. These figures are useful for understanding the calculation and for the practice questions in this book, but never identify a drop factor from the type of infusion alone in real practice. Always read the drop factor actually printed on the giving set packaging in front of you, every time, regardless of what type of set it is or what you used earlier that shift. Using the wrong figure, whether from memory, habit, or assumption based on the fluid being given, is a direct and well recognised cause of rate calculation errors.

The calculation itself takes the volume to be given, converts it into a number of drops using the drop factor, and divides that figure by the time in minutes to give a rate in drops per minute. Written as a formula: volume in mL, multiplied by the drop factor, divided by time in minutes.

Reading the Label

IV PRESCRIPTION	GIVING SET PACKAGING
Fluid: Sod. Chloride 0.9% Volume: 500 mL Duration: 4 hours Route: IV, gravity	Standard Solution Set Drop factor: 20 drops/mL Single use only

What do you notice before calculating anything?

The drop factor is printed directly on the packaging in front of you, exactly where this chapter says to look, rather than assumed from the type of set or fluid. Working it through: convert time to minutes, 4 × 60 = 240. Multiply volume by drop factor: 500 × 20 = 10,000. Divide by time: 10,000 ÷ 240 = 41.67, rounding to approximately 42 drops per minute.

Worked Example 10.3: Drops per Minute with a Standard Giving Set

A patient is prescribed 1 litre of fluid over 8 hours, using a giving set with a drop factor of 20 drops per mL. What is the rate in drops per minute?

Step 1: Convert the volume to mL: 1 litre = 1000 mL.

Step 2: Convert the time to minutes: 8 hours × 60 = 480 minutes.

Step 3: Multiply the volume by the drop factor: 1000 × 20 = 20,000.

Step 4: Divide by the time in minutes: 20,000 ÷ 480 = 41.67.

Step 5: Round to the nearest whole drop, since a fraction of a drop cannot be delivered.

Answer: Set the rate to approximately 42 drops per minute

Worked Example 10.4: Drops per Minute with a Blood Giving Set

A unit of blood, 350 mL, is to be given over 3 hours using a blood giving set with a drop factor of 15 drops per mL. What is the rate in drops per minute?

Step 1: Convert the time to minutes: 3 hours × 60 = 180 minutes.

Step 2: Multiply the volume by the drop factor: 350 × 15 = 5250.

Step 3: Divide by the time in minutes: 5250 ÷ 180 = 29.17.

Step 4: Round to the nearest whole drop.

Answer: Set the rate to approximately 29 drops per minute

Why Rounding Direction Matters Here

Drops per minute is one of the few calculations in this book where the direction of rounding deserves a specific comment. A drop cannot be partially delivered, so the figure must be rounded to a whole number, but rounding up versus rounding down produces a genuinely different infusion time over the course of a long infusion, and for most routine infusions the standard mathematical rounding rule, round to the nearest whole number, is appropriate and safe. For fluids or medications with a narrow safety margin, local policy may specify rounding down rather than to the nearest whole number, to avoid ever infusing faster than intended. Where local policy and standard rounding conflict, local policy takes precedence, and this is worth confirming for high-risk infusions specifically.

Key Points

- Pump rates in mL per hour are calculated as total volume divided by total time in hours.
- Drop factor states how many drops of a specific giving set equal 1 mL, and must be read from the packaging every time, never assumed.
- Drops per minute equals volume in mL multiplied by the drop factor, divided by time in minutes.
- Always convert time to minutes before calculating a drops per minute rate.
- Round drops per minute to a whole number, and check local policy for high-risk infusions where rounding direction may be specified.

CHAPTER 11

Infusion Time and Volume Calculations

Chapter 10 covered the two core IV rate formulas, mL per hour and drops per minute. This chapter uses the same underlying relationship between volume, rate, and time to answer a different set of questions that come up constantly in real practice: how much longer will this infusion run, how much volume is left in the bag, what time will it finish, and how do you convert between a pump rate and a drop rate when handing over care or troubleshooting a gravity set. None of this requires new formulas. It requires being comfortable rearranging the same relationship to solve for whichever quantity is missing.

The Same Three Quantities, Rearranged

Every IV rate calculation involves exactly three quantities: total volume, total time, and rate. Chapter 10 showed how to find rate when volume and time are known, dividing volume by time. The same relationship rearranges to find either of the other two quantities, depending on which two are known and which one is missing. If you know the rate and the time, multiplying them gives the volume. If you know the rate and the volume, dividing the volume by the rate gives the time.

This is worth stating explicitly because students sometimes treat these as three separate things to memorise, when they are really one relationship viewed from three different angles. Once you are confident with the reasoning rather than a fixed formula, it does not matter which two quantities a question gives you, you can always find the third.

Worked Example 11.1: Finding Remaining Time

A 1 litre bag is running at 125 mL per hour. 600 mL has already infused. How much longer will the infusion take to complete?

Step 1: Find the volume remaining: 1000 mL – 600 mL = 400 mL.

Step 2: Time equals volume divided by rate: 400 ÷ 125.

Step 3: 400 ÷ 125 = 3.2 hours.

Step 4: Convert 0.2 hours to minutes: 0.2 × 60 = 12 minutes.

Answer: The infusion will take a further 3 hours and 12 minutes

Worked Example 11.2: Finding Volume Infused Over Elapsed Time

An infusion has been running at 80 mL per hour for 2 hours and 30 minutes. How much volume has been given?

Step 1: Convert the elapsed time to a decimal number of hours: 2 hours 30 minutes = 2.5 hours.

Step 2: Volume equals rate multiplied by time: 80 × 2.5.

Step 3: 80 × 2.5 = 200.

Answer: 200 mL has been infused

Working Out a Completion Time

A very common practical question is not how long an infusion will take, but what time it will actually finish, which requires adding the calculated duration onto the current clock time. This step is not mathematically complex, but it is a place where errors creep in, particularly around the hour changing or crossing midnight, so it is worth treating as a deliberate final step rather than something to do in your head while distracted.

Worked Example 11.3: Calculating Completion Time

An infusion is started at 14:40 and is calculated to take 3 hours and 12 minutes to complete. What time will it finish?

Step 1: Add the hours first: 14:40 + 3 hours = 17:40.

Step 2: Add the remaining minutes: 17:40 + 12 minutes = 17:52.

Answer: The infusion will finish at 17:52

Converting Between mL per Hour and Drops per Minute

Occasionally you will need to convert a rate already expressed in mL per hour into drops per minute, for example when a prescribed pump rate needs to be delivered on a gravity set because a pump is not available. This is simply the drops per minute formula from Chapter 10, applied to an hourly rate rather than a total volume, remembering to convert the hourly rate down to a per-minute basis.

Worked Example 11.4: Converting a Pump Rate to Drops per Minute

A pump rate of 84 mL per hour needs to be delivered using a gravity giving set with a drop factor of 20 drops per mL. What is the equivalent rate in drops per minute?

Step 1: Multiply the hourly volume by the drop factor: 84 × 20 = 1680 drops per hour.

Step 2: Divide by 60 to convert to drops per minute: 1680 ÷ 60 = 28.

Answer: Set the gravity infusion to 28 drops per minute

A Practical Habit: Checking the Bag, Not Just the Number

Every calculation in this chapter assumes the numbers you started with, the volume in the bag and the rate on the pump or clamp, are accurate at the moment you check them. In practice, this means physically checking the volume remaining in the bag against what the calculation predicts, at reasonable intervals during a long infusion, rather than trusting the pump display or a mental estimate alone. A discrepancy between the expected and actual volume remaining is a useful early signal that the programmed rate does not match what was intended, or that the set has been altered since it was started, and it is worth investigating as soon as it is noticed.

It is worth being precise about what this check does and does not tell you. A pump will keep moving fluid out of the bag at its programmed rate regardless of whether that fluid is actually reaching the bloodstream, so the volume remaining in the bag matching the calculation does not, on its own, confirm that the cannula site is healthy or that the fluid is being delivered where intended. Checking bag volume against the calculation is a check on the rate and the fluid balance, and it should sit alongside, not instead of, a proper assessment of the patient and the cannula site itself.

Key Points

- Volume, time, and rate are one relationship viewed three ways: rate is volume over time, volume is rate times time, and time is volume over rate.
- Always find the volume remaining before calculating remaining time, do not use the original total volume.
- Add durations onto clock time as a deliberate final step, watching carefully for the hour changing.
- Converting mL per hour to drops per minute uses the same drop factor formula from Chapter 10, applied to an hourly volume.
- Physically check actual volume remaining against the calculated expectation during long infusions, discrepancies are an early warning sign.

CHAPTER 12

High-Risk IV Medications: Why These Need Extra Checks

Every calculation method in this book applies equally to every drug, but not every drug carries the same consequence if a calculation goes wrong. A small error in a dose of an antibiotic with a wide margin of safety may have no clinically meaningful effect at all. The same size of error in a small number of specific medications can cause serious harm or death within minutes. This chapter is not about new arithmetic. It is about recognising which medications fall into that second category and understanding why standard practice around them is deliberately more cautious than usual.

What Makes a Medication High-Risk

A medication is generally considered high-risk, sometimes called high-alert, when it has a narrow margin between an effective dose and a harmful one, when errors are more likely to cause serious harm even if they occur infrequently, or when the effect of an error cannot easily be reversed once it has been given. Concentrated potassium chloride, insulin, opioids, anticoagulants such as heparin, and vasoactive drugs such as inotropes and vasopressors are commonly cited examples, alongside chemotherapy agents and neuromuscular blocking drugs.

None of these drugs require a different calculation method from the ones already covered in this book. What differs is the acceptable margin for error and, correspondingly, the checking process wrapped around the calculation before it reaches the patient.

Independent Double-Checking

Follow your local policy on which medications require an independent second check, since this varies between organisations and clinical areas, and high-risk IV medications are frequently included. Where a second check is required, the word independent is doing real work in that phrase. An effective double-check means a second person calculates the dose separately, from the original prescription, without seeing the first person's working, and compares their answer at the end. A second person simply watching the first person's calculation and agreeing that it looks right is not an independent check, it is a much weaker safeguard, because it relies on the second person spotting an error in someone else's reasoning rather than generating an independent answer to compare against.

This distinction matters because errors that occur inside someone's reasoning, a wrong assumption about units, a formula applied incorrectly, are often invisible to that same person when they check their own work again, and are also easy for an observer to miss if they are simply following along rather than calculating independently themselves.

Smart Pumps and Dose Error Reduction

Many infusion pumps now include a drug library with pre-set concentration limits and dose range alerts, sometimes referred to as dose error reduction software. These systems can flag a programmed rate that falls outside an expected range for a specific drug, adding a further layer of protection beyond the calculation and the double-check. It is worth understanding what these systems do and do not do. They check a programmed rate against a pre-set range, they do not verify that the underlying calculation was performed correctly in the first place, and they do not replace the need for an accurate calculation or, where required by local policy, an independent check. A rate that is wrong but happens to fall within the software's alert range will not be flagged.

Titrated Infusions: Doses That Change with Response

Some high-risk infusions, particularly vasoactive drugs used in critical care, are prescribed not as a fixed rate but as a dose per kilogram of body weight per minute, adjusted up or down according to the patient's ongoing response, for example blood pressure. This is a preview of the weight-based reasoning covered fully in Part Five, but it is worth introducing here because it illustrates exactly why these infusions are treated with such caution: every time the dose is titrated, a new pump rate has to be calculated, which means every titration is a fresh opportunity for a calculation error, not just a single one at the start of the infusion.

Worked Example 12.1: Converting a Titrated Dose to a Pump Rate

A patient weighing 70 kg is prescribed an infusion at 0.1 micrograms per kg per minute. The infusion bag contains 4 mg of drug in 50 mL. What rate, in mL per hour, should the pump be set to?

Step 1: Calculate the dose per minute for this patient: 0.1 micrograms × 70 kg = 7 micrograms per minute.

Step 2: Convert to a dose per hour: 7 × 60 = 420 micrograms per hour.

Step 3: Convert the bag concentration to micrograms per mL: 4 mg = 4000 micrograms, and 4000 ÷ 50 mL = 80 micrograms per mL.

Step 4: Divide the hourly dose by the concentration to find the rate: 420 ÷ 80 = 5.25 mL per hour.

Answer: Set the pump to 5.25 mL per hour

Recognising When Something Looks Wrong

A practical habit worth building specifically for high-risk infusions is having a rough sense of the typical range a rate should fall in, so that a result well outside that range prompts a recheck before administration rather than after. This is the same sense-check principle introduced in Chapter 4 for tablet counts, applied here to a context where the consequence of missing an error is considerably higher. If a titrated infusion calculation produces a rate of 50 mL per hour when similar patients are typically around 5 mL per hour, that tenfold difference is far more likely to represent a missed decimal point or a unit conversion error than a genuinely unusual clinical picture, and it is worth working back through the calculation before proceeding, not after.

Key Points

- High-risk medications do not require different maths, they require a smaller acceptable margin for error and more rigorous checking.
- An effective independent double-check means calculating separately from the original prescription, not simply reviewing someone else's working.
- Smart pump dose error reduction software checks a programmed rate against a preset range, it does not verify the calculation itself.
- Titrated infusions require a fresh calculation at every dose change, multiplying the opportunities for error over the course of treatment.
- A result far outside the typical expected range for a high-risk infusion should always be rechecked before, not after, administration.

CHAPTER 13

Practice Set 3: IV Flow Rates and High-Risk Infusions

This set covers Part Four: pump rates, drops per minute, rearranging volume, time, and rate, and the extra checking considerations that apply to high-risk infusions. Fourteen questions this time. As with Practice Set 2, one question asks you to evaluate a situation rather than calculate a number. Work through all fourteen questions before turning to the Solutions section at the back of the book.

Question 1 · Foundation

A patient is prescribed 1.5 litres of fluid over 12 hours via an infusion pump. What rate, in mL per hour, should the pump be set to?

Question 2 · Foundation

A 250 mL bag is prescribed over 2 hours, using a standard giving set with a drop factor of 20 drops per mL. What is the rate in drops per minute?

Question 3 · Foundation

An infusion is running at 100 mL per hour from a 1 litre bag. 350 mL has infused so far. How much longer will it take to complete?

Question 4 · Clinical Application

An infusion started at 09:15 is calculated to run for 4 hours and 45 minutes. What time will it complete?

Question 5 · Clinical Application

A pump rate of 60 mL per hour needs to be converted to a gravity infusion using a giving set with a drop factor of 20 drops per mL. What is the equivalent rate in drops per minute?

Question 6 · Clinical Application

A patient weighing 80 kg is prescribed an infusion at 0.05 micrograms per kg per minute. The bag contains 5 mg in 50 mL. What rate, in mL per hour, should the pump be set to?

Question 7 · Challenge

A unit of blood, 300 mL, is prescribed over 2 hours using a blood giving set with a drop factor of 15 drops per mL. What is the rate in drops per minute?

Question 8 · Challenge: Evaluate the Situation

A nurse calculates a titrated vasopressor rate and, being confident in the answer, asks a colleague to glance at the number on the pump screen and confirm it looks reasonable before starting the infusion. The colleague agrees it looks fine. Has an appropriate independent double-check taken place?

Question 9 · Foundation

A patient is prescribed 2 litres of fluid over 16 hours via a pump. What rate, in mL per hour, should the pump be set to?

Question 10 · Foundation

An infusion is running at 60 mL per hour. How long will it take to give 180 mL?

Question 11 · Clinical Application

A 200 mL bag is prescribed over 90 minutes using a giving set with a drop factor of 20 drops per mL, as stated on the packaging. What is the rate in drops per minute?

Question 12 · Clinical Application

An infusion running at 90 mL per hour has had 450 mL infused from a 1 litre bag. What time will it finish if it started at 08:20?

Question 13 · Challenge

A patient weighing 65 kg is prescribed a titrated infusion at 0.08 micrograms per kg per minute. The bag contains 4 mg in 40 mL. What rate, in mL per hour, should the pump be set to?

Question 14 · Challenge

A calculated titrated infusion rate comes out at 45 mL per hour, where similar patients on this drug typically run at 4 to 6 mL per hour. What should the nurse do before programming the pump?

How Did You Do?

By this point in the book, the volume, time, and rate relationship from Chapter 11 should be starting to feel as automatic as the dose required over dose available formula from Part Two. If it does not yet, it is worth returning to Chapter 10 and Chapter 11 before moving on, because Part Five builds weight-based and paediatric dosing directly on top of this same reasoning, adding one further variable, body weight, into a relationship you should already trust.

PART V

Weight-Based and Paediatric Calculations

CHAPTER 14

Weight-Based Dose Calculations

Many medications are prescribed not as a fixed dose for every adult, but as an amount per kilogram of the patient's body weight, because the right dose of many drugs depends on body size. This is especially common in paediatric prescribing, covered in detail in the next two chapters, but it also applies to a range of adult medications, including certain antibiotics, anticoagulants, and chemotherapy agents, where matching the dose to the patient's actual size meaningfully affects both safety and effectiveness.

The calculation itself introduces one new variable, body weight, on top of everything covered so far, but it does not introduce a new kind of reasoning. It simply adds one more multiplication step before the familiar dose required over dose available method takes over.

The Core Weight-Based Formula

A weight-based prescription states a dose per kilogram, for example 5 mg per kg. To find the total dose for a specific patient, multiply the dose per kilogram by the patient's weight in kilograms. This total dose then becomes the dose required in exactly the same tablet, liquid, or injection calculation covered in earlier chapters. Weight-based dosing does not replace those methods, it simply supplies the dose required figure that feeds into them.

Worked Example 14.1: Finding the Total Dose

A patient weighing 62 kg is prescribed a drug at 5 mg per kg. What is the total dose required?

Step 1: Identify the dose per kg: 5 mg per kg.

Step 2: Identify the patient's weight: 62 kg.

Step 3: Multiply: 5 × 62 = 310.

Answer: The total dose required is 310 mg

Worked Example 14.2: Combining Weight-Based Dosing with a Liquid Calculation

A patient weighing 18 kg is prescribed a drug at 10 mg per kg, available as a suspension of 125 mg in 5 mL. How many mL should be given?

Step 1: Find the total dose: 10 × 18 = 180 mg.

Step 2: This 180 mg is now the dose required for a standard liquid calculation.

Step 3: Dose required: 180 mg. Dose available: 125 mg. Volume: 5 mL.

Step 4: Divide: 180 ÷ 125 = 1.44.

Step 5: Multiply by volume: 1.44 × 5 mL = 7.2 mL.

Answer: Give 7.2 mL

When the Prescribed Amount Is a Daily Dose

Some weight-based prescriptions state a total daily amount, for example 30 mg per kg per day, to be split across several doses over the day rather than given all at once. In this situation, an extra step is needed after finding the total daily dose: dividing that daily total by the number of doses to be given each day, to find the amount for each individual dose.

This is a common source of error, specifically when a student or nurse calculates the total daily amount correctly and then administers that full amount at a single dosing time, rather than dividing it across the number of doses prescribed. Always check carefully whether a weight-based figure refers to a single dose or a daily total, since the two require genuinely different final answers.

Worked Example 14.3: A Daily Dose Divided Across Multiple Administrations

A patient weighing 24 kg is prescribed a drug at 40 mg per kg per day, to be given in three divided doses. What is the amount for each individual dose?

Step 1: Find the total daily dose: 40 × 24 = 960 mg per day.

Step 2: Divide the daily total by the number of doses: 960 ÷ 3.

Step 3: 960 ÷ 3 = 320.

Answer: Give 320 mg per dose, three times a day

Always Use an Accurate, Current Weight in Kilograms

The entire calculation depends on the weight figure being accurate and current. An estimated weight, a weight recorded weeks or months earlier, or a weight recorded in the wrong units and converted incorrectly, all introduce error before the calculation itself even begins. Whenever possible, a patient should be weighed using calibrated scales at the point of prescribing, rather than relying on a self-reported or historical figure, and any weight given in pounds or stones must be converted fully to kilograms, using the method covered in Chapter 3, before it enters a weight-based calculation.

This point matters more than it might first appear, because a weight-based calculation performed with complete arithmetic accuracy is still unsafe if the weight itself was wrong to begin with. Checking the weight is not a separate task from the calculation, it is the first step of it.

Checking Against a Maximum Dose

Many weight-based drugs have a stated maximum single or daily dose, printed in the product literature or local formulary, which exists because for larger patients, a weight-based calculation can occasionally produce a total dose that exceeds the maximum considered safe or necessary, regardless of body weight. Once a weight-based dose has been calculated, it is good practice to check that figure against any stated maximum dose for that drug. This check takes moments and should be treated as a routine final step for any weight-based calculation, not an occasional extra precaution reserved for unusual cases.

It matters exactly what you do if the calculated dose exceeds the stated maximum. The correct response is not to quietly substitute the maximum figure and administer that instead. A calculated dose that exceeds a stated maximum is a signal to stop, do not administer the calculated dose, and escalate: check the prescription carefully, confirm the weight and figures used, and clarify with the prescriber or pharmacist in accordance with local policy before any dose is given. The calculation has told you something important, that the figure needs checking against the prescription, not that you are now authorised to independently decide what dose to give instead. This is a useful general distinction worth carrying through the rest of this book: a calculation answer and an administration decision are not automatically the same thing. Working out what a calculation implies is different from deciding, unilaterally, what to actually give a patient.

Key Points

- Weight-based dosing adds one step, multiplying dose per kg by patient weight in kg, before the standard dose required over dose available method applies.
- Always check carefully whether a stated weight-based figure is a single dose or a total daily dose to be divided.
- Use an accurate, current weight in kilograms, converting from pounds or stones fully before calculating.
- Always check a calculated weight-based dose against any stated maximum dose for that drug.
- A correct calculation built on an inaccurate weight is still an unsafe dose, checking the weight is part of the calculation, not separate from it.

CHAPTER 15

Body Surface Area Calculations

For a small but clinically significant group of medications, principally chemotherapy agents and a limited number of other high-risk drugs, dosing is based not on weight alone but on body surface area, abbreviated BSA. This chapter explains what BSA represents, how it is calculated, and how it feeds into the same dose required over dose available structure used throughout this book. A clear caution belongs at the very start: in real clinical practice, BSA is calculated using a validated calculator, nomogram, or prescribing software, not worked out by hand from a formula under time pressure. The manual method shown here exists to build genuine understanding of where the number comes from, so that the figure a calculator produces makes sense to you rather than being accepted blindly.

Why Body Surface Area Instead of Weight Alone

Body surface area correlates more closely than body weight alone with a number of physiological factors relevant to drug dosing, including metabolic rate and organ function, which is part of why it is preferred for drugs with a narrow safety margin, most notably chemotherapy. Two patients of very different heights can have the same body weight, but quite different surface areas, and for certain drugs this difference matters more to dosing accuracy than weight alone would capture.

BSA is measured in square metres, written as m^2. A typical adult BSA falls roughly in the range of 1.5 to 2.0 m^2, though this varies considerably with height and weight, which is precisely why it needs to be calculated individually for each patient rather than assumed.

Calculating BSA: The Mosteller Formula

Several formulas exist for estimating BSA from height and weight, and the Mosteller formula is one of the most widely used in clinical practice because of its relative simplicity. It states that BSA in square metres equals the square root of height in centimetres multiplied by weight in kilograms, divided by 3600.

Working through this formula by hand reinforces where a BSA figure comes from, but as noted above, real clinical dosing should always use a validated calculator or nomogram to reduce the risk of manual calculation error feeding into a high-risk chemotherapy dose.

Worked Example 15.1: Calculating BSA

A patient is 170 cm tall and weighs 65 kg. Calculate their body surface area using the Mosteller formula.

Step 1: Multiply height by weight: 170 × 65 = 11,050.

Step 2: Divide by 3600: 11,050 ÷ 3600 = 3.0694 (rounded).

Step 3: Take the square root: the square root of 3.0694 is approximately 1.75.

Answer: The patient's BSA is approximately 1.75 m^2

Applying BSA to a Dose Calculation

A BSA-based prescription states a dose per square metre, for example 100 mg per m^2. Once BSA has been established, usually via a validated calculator rather than the manual method above, the total dose is found by multiplying the dose per m^2 by the patient's BSA, exactly as a weight-based dose is found by multiplying dose per kg by weight. This total dose then feeds into the same tablet, liquid, or injection calculation covered in earlier chapters.

Worked Example 15.2: Finding a BSA-Based Total Dose

A patient has a BSA of 1.75 m^2 and is prescribed a drug at 100 mg per m^2. What is the total dose required?

Step 1: Identify the dose per m^2: 100 mg.

Step 2: Identify the patient's BSA: 1.75 m^2.

Step 3: Multiply: 100 × 1.75 = 175.

Answer: The total dose required is 175 mg

Why This Area Demands Particular Caution

BSA-based dosing sits at the intersection of several risk factors covered separately elsewhere in this book: it is most often used for chemotherapy, a drug category with an extremely narrow margin between an effective and a harmful dose, it depends on an intermediate calculated figure, BSA itself, which introduces an additional opportunity for error before the dose calculation even begins, and it typically involves multiple steps chained together, height and weight into BSA, BSA into total dose, total dose into a volume or infusion rate.

For exactly these reasons, chemotherapy dosing in real clinical practice is subject to some of the most rigorous checking processes of any medication category, typically involving independent double-checking at multiple stages, validated calculation software rather than manual arithmetic, and pharmacy verification before a dose is prepared. Understanding the underlying maths, as this chapter aims to do, supports engaging meaningfully with that checking process, rather than treating a computer-generated figure as something to accept without comprehension.

Key Points

- Body surface area, measured in m^2, is used for drugs where it predicts an effective and safe dose more reliably than weight alone, principally chemotherapy.
- The Mosteller formula estimates BSA as the square root of height in cm multiplied by weight in kg, divided by 3600.
- A BSA-based total dose is found by multiplying dose per m^2 by the patient's BSA, then used in the standard dose required over dose available method.
- Real clinical practice calculates BSA using a validated calculator or nomogram, not manual arithmetic, due to the high stakes involved.

- BSA-based chemotherapy dosing warrants particularly rigorous independent checking, given the narrow safety margin and multiple calculation steps involved.

CHAPTER 16

Paediatric-Specific Safety Considerations

Every calculation method covered in this book applies to paediatric patients just as it does to adults, weight-based dosing, liquid and injection formulas, unit conversions. What changes in paediatric practice is not the arithmetic but the margin for error, and this chapter focuses specifically on why that margin is smaller, where paediatric-specific mistakes tend to occur, and the additional checks that reflect this.

Why Small Errors Matter More in Children

A calculation error of a fixed size has a very different impact depending on the size of the patient it is applied to. An error that adds an extra 50 mg to a dose intended for a 70 kg adult may fall within a wide margin of safety. The same 50 mg error applied to a dose intended for a 5 kg infant represents a proportionally enormous difference, and may far exceed any safe margin at all. This is the core reason paediatric dosing demands particular caution, not because the maths is different, but because paediatric doses are frequently small numbers, close to the level of everyday calculation errors, given to patients with very little physiological reserve to absorb a mistake.

This proportional sensitivity also means that decimal point errors, already identified in Chapter 2 as one of the most dangerous mistakes in any dose calculation, are especially hazardous in paediatric practice, precisely because paediatric doses already routinely involve decimals and small numbers, making a misplaced decimal point harder to visually spot as obviously wrong compared with an adult dose.

Always Use an Accurate, Current, Measured Weight

The point made in Chapter 14 about using an accurate current weight applies with even greater force in paediatric practice, because children's weights change relatively quickly compared with adults, and a weight from a previous admission or an estimated figure can be meaningfully out of date within weeks, not years. Wherever possible, paediatric doses should be calculated using a weight measured on the day, using calibrated scales, rather than a historical or parent-reported figure.

In genuine emergencies where a child cannot be weighed immediately, age-based weight estimation formulas exist and are used specifically for that emergency context, but these are estimates intended to bridge an urgent situation, not a substitute for an actual measured weight in routine, non-emergency dosing.

Reading the Label

PAEDIATRIC PRESCRIPTION	STOCK LABEL
Drug: Amoxicillin Dose: 25 mg/kg/day Weight: 18 kg (today) Divided: three times daily	Amoxicillin Susp. 125 mg in 5 mL SHAKE WELL

What do you notice before calculating anything?

Notice the weight is explicitly marked as taken today, exactly the safeguard this chapter has been building toward, rather than a figure carried over from a previous visit. Working through it: total daily dose 25 × 18 = 450 mg, divided by three doses = 150 mg per dose. Applying the standard liquid method: dose required 150 mg, dose available 125 mg, volume 5 mL. 150 ÷ 125 = 1.2, × 5 mL = 6 mL per dose.

Checking Against Both a Weight-Based Range and an Adult Maximum

Paediatric dose references, such as the British National Formulary for Children, typically state a recommended dose per kg alongside a maximum dose that should not be exceeded regardless of weight. This maximum exists because larger children and adolescents, calculated purely on a mg per kg basis, can sometimes produce a total dose that equals or exceeds a standard adult dose, which is rarely the intention. Checking a calculated paediatric dose against both the expected mg per kg range and any stated maximum is a necessary final step, not an optional extra.

Worked Example 16.1: Checking a Calculation Against a Maximum Dose

A 45 kg adolescent is prescribed a drug at 15 mg per kg, with a stated maximum single dose of 600 mg. What should happen next?

Step 1: Calculate the weight-based dose: 15 × 45 = 675 mg.

Step 2: Compare this to the stated maximum single dose of 600 mg.

Step 3: 675 mg exceeds the maximum. This is a signal to stop, not a signal to self-correct.

Answer: Do not administer 675 mg. The calculated dose exceeds the stated maximum of 600 mg, so the prescription and figures used should be checked, and the prescriber or pharmacist contacted in line with local policy before any dose is given.

Formulations, Devices, and Avoiding Misconnection

Paediatric doses are frequently prepared using oral syringes rather than measuring cups or spoons, both for the fine graduation discussed in Chapter 5 and 7, and for safety reasons specific to children, including preventing a young child from independently accessing a full bottle of liquid medication. Many healthcare settings use oral syringes with a design that cannot physically connect to an intravenous line, a deliberate engineering safeguard against a medication intended for oral administration being mistakenly given intravenously, an error with obviously serious consequences.

As with tablets in Chapter 4, paediatric-specific formulations, including specific liquid concentrations designed for smaller doses, should be used in preference to attempting to measure a very small volume from a preparation designed for adult dosing, since the accuracy achievable is directly related to how well the available concentration matches the size of dose actually needed.

Independent Double-Checking in Paediatric Practice

Given the combination of small doses, narrow safety margins, and frequent weight-based calculation, local policy in many organisations extends independent double-checking, as defined in Chapter 12, to paediatric medications more broadly, not only those classed as high-risk in adult practice. Always follow your own organisation's medicines policy on which paediatric medications require a second check, since this is set locally and can vary. The broader point stands regardless of the specific local policy in place: in paediatric care, the checking habits that are reserved for particularly dangerous drugs in adult practice are worth applying more readily, because the patient population itself carries a narrower margin for error across the board.

Key Points

- The same fixed calculation error is proportionally far more dangerous in a small child than in an adult.
- Decimal point errors are especially hazardous in paediatric dosing because paediatric doses already routinely involve small numbers and decimals.
- Always use an accurate, current, measured weight, paediatric weight can change significantly in a short time.
- Check a calculated paediatric dose against both the expected mg per kg range and any stated maximum dose.

- Independent double-checking is commonly required for paediatric medicines; always follow local policy regarding which medications require a second check.

CHAPTER 17

Practice Set 4: Weight-Based, BSA, and Paediatric Dosing

This final practice set covers Part Five: weight-based dosing, body surface area, and the additional safety considerations specific to paediatric practice. Fourteen questions this time. As with the previous two sets, one question asks you to evaluate a scenario rather than calculate a figure. Work through all fourteen questions before turning to the Solutions section at the back of the book.

Question 1 · Foundation

A patient weighing 54 kg is prescribed a drug at 8 mg per kg. What is the total dose required?

Question 2 · Foundation

A child weighing 14 kg is prescribed a drug at 12 mg per kg, available as a suspension of 250 mg in 5 mL. How many mL should be given?

Question 3 · Foundation

A child weighing 20 kg is prescribed a drug at 50 mg per kg per day, in four divided doses. What is the amount for each individual dose?

Question 4 · Clinical Application

Calculate the BSA of a patient who is 160 cm tall and weighs 70 kg, using the Mosteller formula.

Question 5 · Clinical Application

A patient has a BSA of 1.6 m^2 and is prescribed a drug at 75 mg per m^2. What is the total dose required?

Question 6 · Clinical Application

A 40 kg adolescent is prescribed a drug at 20 mg per kg, with a stated maximum single dose of 700 mg. What should happen next?

Question 7 · Challenge

A neonate weighing 3.2 kg is prescribed a drug at 4 mg per kg. What is the total dose required, to one decimal place?

Question 8 · Challenge: Evaluate the Situation

A nurse calculates a paediatric dose using a weight recorded on the patient's admission three weeks earlier, reasoning that a young child's weight would not have changed enough in that time to matter. Is this reasoning sound?

Question 9 · Foundation

A patient weighing 48 kg is prescribed a drug at 10 mg per kg. What is the total dose required?

Question 10 · Foundation

A child weighing 22 kg is prescribed a drug at 15 mg per kg per day, in three divided doses. What is the amount for each individual dose?

Question 11 · Clinical Application

Calculate the BSA of a patient who is 180 cm tall and weighs 85 kg, using the Mosteller formula.

Question 12 · Clinical Application

A patient has a BSA of 1.9 m^2 and is prescribed a drug at 60 mg per m^2. What is the total dose required?

Question 13 · Challenge

A 30 kg child is prescribed a drug at 12 mg per kg, available as a suspension of 250 mg in 5 mL, with a stated maximum single dose of 300 mg. What should happen?

Question 14 · Challenge

A nurse is asked to calculate a chemotherapy dose based on BSA and, being confident with the Mosteller formula, works it out by hand rather than using the ward's validated BSA calculator, to save time. What does Chapter 15 say about this approach?

How Did You Do?

This is the last practice set in the book, and if you have worked through all four sets in order, the questions in this one should have felt less like new material and more like the same handful of ideas, dose required over dose available, accurate units, accurate weight, checking against a sensible range, applied in a new context. That is precisely the outcome this book has been building toward from Chapter 1: not a long list of separate procedures to memorise, but one way of reasoning that adapts to whatever calculation is in front of you. Part Six closes the book by looking directly at how to carry that reasoning into real practice, under real time pressure, without it falling apart.

PART VI

Think, Check and Perform with Confidence

CHAPTER 18

Common Error Patterns and How to Catch Them Before They Reach the Patient

Every chapter in this book has mentioned specific ways calculations go wrong, a missed decimal point here, an unconverted unit there. This chapter draws those scattered warnings together into a single picture, organised around the underlying pattern behind each type of error, and pairs every pattern with a specific, practical way of catching it before it reaches a patient. Knowing that errors happen is not protective on its own. Knowing the shape a specific error tends to take, and having a deliberate habit that catches that shape, is what actually prevents harm.

Pattern One: The Missing or Misplaced Conversion

This is the error covered most extensively in this book, starting in Chapter 3: a dose prescribed in one unit, a stock item labelled in another, and a calculation performed without converting one of them first. It produces answers that are wrong by a clean factor, most often ten or one thousand, which makes it particularly dangerous, because the resulting number often still looks superficially plausible.

The catch for this pattern is the habit introduced in Chapter 3: write out every quantity involved with its unit clearly stated before doing any arithmetic, and check that they match. This single habit, performed consistently, closes off the majority of conversion errors before the calculation itself even begins.

Pattern Two: The Formula Applied Backwards or Incompletely

This pattern covers a range of related mistakes: dividing dose available by dose required instead of the other way around, forgetting to multiply by volume in a liquid calculation, or omitting the final step that finds a rate from a total. These errors usually stem from applying a formula as a memorised sequence of operations rather than as a shorthand for a question genuinely understood, which is precisely why this book has built every method from first principles rather than presenting formulas to be applied mechanically.

The catch here is a version of the sense-check habit introduced in Chapter 4: before accepting a final answer, briefly restate in plain language what the calculation was actually asking, and check the answer against that question directly, rather than checking only that the arithmetic steps were followed correctly.

Worked Example 18.1: Catching a Backwards Formula

A calculation for a patient prescribed 400 mg, with stock available as 200 mg per tablet, is worked as 200 ÷ 400, giving an answer of 0.5. Identify the error and the correct answer.

Step 1: Restate the question in plain language: how many 200 mg tablets are needed to give 400 mg.

Step 2: A dose larger than a single tablet's strength should require more than one tablet, not less.

Step 3: An answer of 0.5 tablets, less than one, immediately conflicts with this plain-language check.

Step 4: The formula was applied backwards. The correct calculation is 400 ÷ 200 = 2.

Answer: The correct answer is 2 tablets. The original calculation had dose required and dose available reversed.

Pattern Three: The Transcription Slip

Not every error happens inside the maths. A perfectly correct calculation can still lead to a wrong dose if a number was copied incorrectly from the prescription chart, misread from a decimal-heavy figure, or entered incorrectly into a pump after being calculated correctly on paper. This pattern is easy to overlook because it feels like it belongs to documentation rather than calculation, but from the patient's perspective the outcome is identical to a genuine arithmetic error.

The catch is to treat the transfer of a number from one place to another, chart to working, working to pump, as a distinct step worth its own check, reading the figure back against its original source immediately before it is acted upon, rather than assuming that because a number was correct a moment ago it is still correct now.

Pattern Four: Interruption and Fatigue

Drug calculations are frequently performed in environments that are not designed for careful arithmetic, mid-shift, standing at a busy medication trolley, with frequent interruptions from colleagues, call bells, and competing demands. Interruption during a calculation is one of the most well documented contributors to medication error generally, not because any individual interruption is long, but because resuming a partially completed calculation after a break in concentration is a well known point where a step gets skipped, repeated, or misremembered.

Where possible, the practical response is to protect a short, uninterrupted window for calculation itself, even a minute or two, rather than attempting to complete or resume a calculation while simultaneously responding to something else. If interrupted partway through, the safest response is to restart the calculation from the beginning rather than trying to recall exactly which step had been reached.

Pattern Five: Trusting the Answer Because It Came from a Machine

Calculators, smart pumps, and prescribing software all reduce the likelihood of certain kinds of errors, but they introduce a different risk in exchange: a tendency to trust an output simply because it was machine generated, sometimes called automation bias. A calculator will confidently return an answer to whatever numbers are entered into it, including numbers that were themselves entered incorrectly, and a smart pump alert range, as covered in Chapter 12, only checks a programmed rate against a preset boundary, it does not verify that the underlying reasoning was sound.

The catch for this pattern is the sense-check habit that has run through this entire book, applied specifically to machine-generated answers rather than only to manual ones. A number produced by a calculator or a pump deserves the same brief plausibility check as a number worked out by hand: does this fall within a range that makes clinical sense, and does it answer the actual question that was asked.

Key Points

- Missing or misplaced unit conversions are caught by writing out every quantity with its unit before calculating, and checking that units match.
- A backwards or incomplete formula is caught by restating the question in plain language and checking the answer against it directly.
- Transcription errors are caught by treating every transfer of a number as its own checkable step, not an assumed continuation of a previous correct figure.
- Interruption during a calculation is a recognised risk factor. When interrupted, restart the calculation rather than trying to resume from memory.
- A machine-generated answer deserves the same plausibility check as a manually calculated one, automation does not remove the need for clinical judgement.

CHAPTER 19

Double-Checking Strategies That Actually Work

Almost every nursing student is told to check their work, and almost no one is told specifically how to check in a way that actually catches errors, as opposed to simply re-reading the same steps and confirming, unsurprisingly, that they still look the same. This chapter is about the difference between those two things, and about specific checking strategies that genuinely add protection rather than just adding time.

Why Re-Reading Your Own Work Rarely Catches Errors

If a calculation contains an error because of a flawed piece of reasoning, for example forgetting that a value needed converting, or misremembering which way round a formula goes, re-reading the same working from the same starting assumptions will very often reproduce the same flawed reasoning and confirm the same wrong answer. This is not a failure of effort or attention, it is simply how checking works when it follows the identical mental path as the original calculation. The error is invisible from that path because the path itself is what generated it.

Genuinely effective checking requires taking a different route to the answer, one that does not depend on the same assumption being correct twice. The strategies in this chapter are all, in different ways, methods of taking a different route.

Strategy One: Independent Recalculation

This is the gold standard, introduced in Chapter 12 for high-risk medications, and it works precisely because a second person, starting from the original prescription without seeing the first person's working, is not vulnerable to the first person's specific error in reasoning. Two independent calculations that agree provide strong evidence the answer is correct. Two independent calculations that disagree immediately flag that something needs re-examining, before either figure is acted on.

Where a genuinely independent second person is not available or not required by local policy for a lower-risk medication, the remaining strategies in this chapter offer a way of building some of the same protection into a single-person check.

Strategy Two: Working Backwards from the Answer

Rather than re-reading the forward calculation, take the final answer and use it to work back toward the original figures. This uses the same underlying relationship but in reverse, which is a genuinely different mental operation from repeating the forward steps, and it will reliably expose an error that the forward re-reading would miss.

Worked Example 19.1: Checking by Working Backwards

A calculation gives 2 tablets for a prescribed dose of 500 mg, using 250 mg tablets. Check this answer by working backwards.

Step 1: Take the answer, 2 tablets, and the tablet strength, 250 mg.

Step 2: Multiply forward: 2 tablets × 250 mg = 500 mg.

Step 3: Compare this to the originally prescribed dose of 500 mg.

Step 4: The two figures match.

Answer: The calculation checks out, 2 tablets of 250 mg correctly delivers the prescribed 500 mg

---

Strategy Three: Estimating Before Calculating Precisely

Before working through the exact arithmetic, take a moment to estimate roughly what the answer should be, using rounded, easy numbers. If a patient needs roughly 500 mg and the tablets are roughly 250 mg each, the answer should be roughly 2, without doing any precise arithmetic at all. Once the precise calculation is complete, compare it against this rough estimate. If the precise answer and the rough estimate are wildly different, something has gone wrong somewhere, most likely a decimal point or unit conversion error, and it is worth finding before proceeding.

This strategy is fast, requires no extra tools, and specifically catches the class of error, decimal and unit errors, most likely to produce a dangerously large or small final answer.

Strategy Four: Solving It a Different Way

Where a calculation can genuinely be approached through more than one valid method, for example converting a ratio strength to mg per mL before multiplying, versus setting up a direct proportion, solving it once each way and comparing the results is a strong check, because an error specific to one method is unlikely to appear identically in a completely different method. This will not always be practical under time pressure, but it is a particularly good habit to build during study and practice, when there is no clinical urgency, so that the underlying flexibility becomes available later when it matters most.

Strategy Five: Explaining the Calculation Out Loud

Putting a calculation into spoken words, either to a colleague or simply to yourself, forces a level of explicit reasoning that silent mental arithmetic can skip past. Gaps in reasoning that feel fine when thought quickly and silently often become obvious the moment they need to be said aloud in a coherent sentence. This is a genuinely useful strategy even alone, and it is one of the reasons an effective independent double-check often includes a brief verbal walk-through of the reasoning, not just a comparison of final numbers.

Key Points

- Re-reading your own calculation rarely catches an error, because it follows the same reasoning path that produced the error in the first place.
- Independent recalculation by a second person, from the original prescription, is the strongest available check.
- Working backwards from the final answer to the original figures uses a genuinely different mental operation than re-reading forward.
- A rough estimate calculated before the precise answer catches large errors, particularly decimal and unit conversion mistakes.
- Explaining a calculation aloud forces explicit reasoning and often exposes gaps that silent checking misses.

CHAPTER 20

Calculation Confidence Under Pressure

Chapter 1 opened this book by separating calculation ability from calculation anxiety, and by explaining that the two need different solutions. Nineteen chapters later, the calculation ability side of that equation should be considerably stronger than it was at the start. This final full chapter turns back to the second half of the problem directly: how to hold onto that ability when it is tested under real pressure, whether that pressure comes from an exam hall or a busy ward.

What Pressure Actually Does

Time pressure, being observed, and the fear of consequences all draw on the same limited mental resource, working memory, that calculation itself depends on. This is why a calculation that feels entirely manageable in quiet, unhurried practice can suddenly feel much harder in an exam hall or at a medication trolley with a queue of patients waiting, even though the arithmetic involved has not changed at all. Understanding this is not an excuse or a reason to expect to perform worse under pressure, it is the reason the specific techniques in this chapter exist, because they are designed to reduce how much working memory the pressure itself consumes, leaving more available for the calculation.

In an Exam: Concrete Techniques

Read the entire question once before writing anything down, resisting the urge to start calculating from the first number that appears. Many calculation questions are deliberately structured with information presented out of order, or with an irrelevant figure included specifically to test whether it gets used incorrectly. Reading the whole question first, then writing out every relevant quantity with its unit clearly stated, exactly as recommended in

Chapter 3, externalises the information onto paper and frees up working memory that would otherwise be spent holding numbers in your head while also trying to reason about them.

Estimate before calculating precisely, as covered in Chapter 19. A quick rough estimate, formed in seconds, gives you an anchor to check the final answer against, and this anchor is genuinely reassuring under pressure, because it means you are not relying purely on trust in a sequence of steps performed quickly and under stress. If your precise answer lands close to your rough estimate, that is a real, evidence-based reason for confidence in that specific answer, not a vague reassurance.

If a particular question is not coming together, move on and return to it rather than allowing it to consume time and mental energy that the rest of the exam also needs. A calculation question left blank and returned to with a clearer head after other questions is very often solved quickly the second time, precisely because the specific pressure of being stuck on it has been temporarily removed.

On the Ward: A Different Kind of Pressure

Clinical pressure differs from exam pressure in an important way: it is rarely just about the calculation itself, it is compounded by interruption, by the presence of colleagues or patients, and sometimes by a reluctance to be seen taking time or asking a question. Chapter 18 already covered why interruption is a genuine risk factor for calculation errors, not simply an inconvenience, and the practical response remains the same, protecting a short uninterrupted window wherever possible, and restarting rather than resuming a calculation broken by an interruption.

The reluctance to be seen taking time deserves addressing directly, because it drives some of the most avoidable errors in real practice. A nurse who feels pressure to appear fast and confident may rush a calculation, skip a check they know is appropriate, or hesitate to ask a colleague to verify a figure, purely to avoid seeming uncertain. Every practising nurse, at every level of experience, checks calculations, asks a colleague to verify a dose, and takes a moment to work through a figure carefully. This is not a sign of weakness or inexperience, it is standard, expected professional practice, and framing it as anything else is itself part of what drives calculation anxiety in the first place.

If You Go Blank

Every person who works with numbers under pressure occasionally experiences a moment where a calculation that should be straightforward suddenly will not come together, the steps blur, and nothing feels certain. When this happens, the most effective response is not to push harder along the same mental path, but to stop, take a breath, and return to the most basic version of the question, restated in plain language, exactly as recommended for catching backwards formulas in Chapter 18. What is actually being asked here, in the simplest possible terms. Very often, rebuilding the calculation slowly from that plain-language starting point succeeds where trying to force the original, half-formed attempt did not.

If that does not resolve things, asking a colleague for a second opinion or a fresh calculation is always the appropriate next step, and never a mark against your competence. Safe medication practice uses several layers of protection, including individual calculation checks, independent double-checking where required by local policy, pharmacy verification, and dose error reduction software. When a calculation remains uncertain after checking it yourself, stop and seek an appropriate second opinion in line with local policy. Asking for help at the moment you need it is not a departure from safe practice. It is safe practice.

Key Points

- Time pressure and observation draw on the same working memory that calculation itself needs, which is why familiar calculations can feel harder under pressure.

- In an exam, read the full question first, write out quantities with units, estimate before calculating precisely, and move on from a stuck question rather than losing time to it.
- On the ward, protect a short uninterrupted window for a calculation, and restart rather than resume one broken by an interruption.
- Checking a calculation or asking a colleague to verify a dose is standard professional practice at every level of experience, not a sign of weakness.
- If you go blank, stop and restate the question in the simplest possible plain language, and ask for a second opinion if that does not resolve it.

CHAPTER 21

Mock Assessment: Final Challenge

This final challenge draws on every part of the book, numeracy, tablets and liquids, injections and unit-based drugs, IV rates, and weight-based and paediatric dosing, in no particular order. Treat it as a genuine exam: work through all twenty questions on paper, under exam-like conditions if you can manage it, before turning to the Solutions section at the back of the book. Note your confidence in each answer as you go. If a particular question exposes a gap, the chapter it draws on is noted alongside the question, so you know exactly where to return.

Question 1 · Foundation (Chapter 4)

A patient is prescribed 900 mg of a drug. Tablets are available in 300 mg strength. How many tablets should be given?

Question 2 · Foundation (Chapter 5)

A patient is prescribed 300 mg of a drug, available as 100 mg in 4 mL. How many mL should be given?

Question 3 · Foundation (Chapter 3)

A prescription states 0.4 mg. Stock is labelled in micrograms. Convert 0.4 mg to micrograms.

Question 4 · Foundation (Chapter 7)

A patient is prescribed 60 mg of a drug by injection, supplied as 100 mg in 2 mL. How many mL should be drawn up, and which syringe size is most appropriate?

Question 5 · Clinical Application (Chapter 8)

A patient is prescribed a heparin bolus of 2000 units, supplied as 5000 units in 5 mL. How many mL should be given?

Question 6 · Clinical Application (Chapter 10)

A patient is prescribed 1.2 litres of fluid over 10 hours via a pump. What rate, in mL per hour, should the pump be set to?

Question 7 · Clinical Application (Chapter 10)

A 500 mL bag is prescribed over 4 hours using a standard giving set with a drop factor of 20 drops per mL. What is the rate in drops per minute?

Question 8 · Clinical Application (Chapter 11)

An infusion running at 150 mL per hour from a 1 litre bag has had 900 mL infused. How much longer will it take to complete?

Question 9 · Clinical Application (Chapter 14)

A patient weighing 58 kg is prescribed a drug at 6 mg per kg. What is the total dose required?

Question 10 · Challenge (Chapter 15)

Calculate the BSA of a patient who is 175 cm tall and weighs 80 kg, using the Mosteller formula.

Question 11 · Challenge (Chapter 16)

A 50 kg adolescent is prescribed a drug at 18 mg per kg, with a stated maximum single dose of 800 mg. What should happen next?

Question 12 · Challenge (Chapters 18 and 19)

A calculation for a patient prescribed 240 mg, using a stock strength of 80 mg per tablet, is worked as 80 ÷ 240, giving 0.33. A rough estimate suggested the answer should be around 3 tablets. What does this tell you, and what is the correct answer?

Question 13 · Foundation (Chapter 3)

Convert 2.4 g to mg.

Question 14 · Foundation (Chapter 2)

How many grams of drug are contained in 80 mL of a 2.5% w/v solution?

Question 15 · Clinical Application (Chapter 5)

A patient is prescribed 450 mg, available as a suspension of 150 mg in 5 mL. How many mL should be given?

Question 16 · Clinical Application (Chapter 7)

A patient is prescribed 45 mg by injection, supplied as 60 mg in 3 mL. How many mL should be drawn up?

Question 17 · Clinical Application (Chapter 11)

An infusion running at 75 mL per hour has had 300 mL infused from a 750 mL bag. How much longer will it take to complete?

Question 18 · Challenge (Chapter 8)

A patient is prescribed a heparin bolus of 1500 units, and the nurse checks the vial, finding it labelled 5000 units in 5 mL. How many mL should be given?

Question 19 · Challenge (Chapters 14 and 16)

A 42 kg child is prescribed a drug at 16 mg per kg, with a stated maximum single dose of 600 mg. What should happen?

Question 20 · Challenge (Chapters 19 and 20)

Midway through a calculation, a nurse is interrupted by a call bell. On returning, they are unsure whether they had already converted the prescribed dose to mg or not, and the figure in front of them could be read either way. What is the safest next step?

Closing Note

If you worked through this exam with steady, unhurried confidence, checking your own reasoning along the way rather than hoping the arithmetic would simply work out, that is exactly the outcome this book set out to build from its very first page. The goal was never to make every calculation trivial. Real clinical calculations will still occasionally be unfamiliar, will still occasionally be given under pressure, and will still occasionally need a second opinion, and all of that is entirely normal. What should feel different now is your relationship to that uncertainty: not a source of dread, but a familiar situation you already know exactly how to handle, one step, one unit, one check at a time.

CHAPTER 22

Mock Assessment: Foundation to Challenge

This second mock assessment gives you one more full pass across the entire book, structured slightly differently from Chapter 21. Questions are grouped explicitly by tier, Foundation first, then Clinical Application, then Challenge, so you can gauge not just whether you get the right answer but at what level of difficulty your confidence starts to waver. Work through all of it on paper before turning to the Solutions section at the back of the book.

Question 1 · Foundation (Chapter 4)

A patient is prescribed 450 mg. Tablets are available in 150 mg strength. How many tablets should be given?

Question 2 · Foundation (Chapter 3)

Convert 1500 micrograms to mg.

Question 3 · Foundation (Chapter 2)

How many grams of drug are contained in 60 mL of a 5% w/v solution?

Question 4 · Foundation (Chapter 5)

A patient is prescribed 200 mg, available as 100 mg in 5 mL. How many mL should be given?

Question 5 · Foundation (Chapter 3)

A patient weighs 9 stone 6 pounds. Convert this to kilograms, to one decimal place.

Question 6 · Clinical Application (Chapter 7)

A patient is prescribed 25 mg by injection, supplied as 50 mg in 2 mL. How many mL should be drawn up?

Question 7 · Clinical Application (Chapter 8)

A patient is prescribed a heparin bolus of 3000 units, supplied as 10,000 units in 10 mL. How many mL should be given?

Question 8 · Clinical Application (Chapter 10)

A patient is prescribed 1 litre over 6 hours via pump. What rate, in mL per hour, should the pump be set to?

Question 9 · Clinical Application (Chapter 10)

A 300 mL bag is prescribed over 3 hours using a giving set with a drop factor stated on the packaging as 20 drops per mL. What is the rate in drops per minute?

Question 10 · Clinical Application (Chapter 14)

A patient weighing 70 kg is prescribed a drug at 4 mg per kg. What is the total dose required?

Question 11 · Clinical Application (Chapter 15)

Calculate the BSA of a patient who is 165 cm tall and weighs 60 kg, using the Mosteller formula.

Question 12 · Clinical Application (Chapter 16)

A child weighing 16 kg is prescribed a drug at 25 mg per kg per day, in two divided doses. What is the amount for each individual dose?

Question 13 · Challenge (Chapters 8 and 12)

A nurse is asked to draw up 8 units of a U-100 insulin. No insulin syringe is available, so they calculate 8 ÷ 100 = 0.08 mL and draw this up using a standard 1 mL syringe. Identify every issue with this approach, not just the arithmetic.

Question 14 · Challenge (Chapters 14 and 16)

A 38 kg child is prescribed a drug at 22 mg per kg, with a stated maximum single dose of 750 mg. The calculated dose exceeds the maximum. What should the nurse do?

Question 15 · Challenge (Chapters 18 and 19)

A calculation for a patient prescribed 320 mg, using a stock strength of 80 mg per tablet, is worked as 80 ÷ 320, giving 0.25. A rough estimate suggested the answer should be around 4 tablets. What does the mismatch tell you, and what is the correct answer?

Question 16 · Foundation (Chapter 3)

Convert 3.6 g to mg.

Question 17 · Foundation (Chapter 2)

How many grams of drug are contained in 150 mL of a 1% w/v solution?

Question 18 · Clinical Application (Chapter 11)

An infusion started at 11:05 is calculated to run for 5 hours and 20 minutes. What time will it complete?

Question 19 · Clinical Application (Chapter 7)

A patient is prescribed 8 mg by injection, supplied as 20 mg in 2 mL. How many mL should be drawn up, and which syringe size is most appropriate?

Question 20 · Challenge (Chapters 8 and 16)

A nurse preparing an insulin dose for a child notices the insulin pen is labelled 200 units per mL, having previously only worked with U-100 insulin as an adult nurse. The prescription states the dose in units. What should the nurse do?

Closing Note

Twenty questions, three tiers, and by this point in the book, hopefully very few surprises in the reasoning required to answer them. That repetition is the point. If you found the Foundation questions close to automatic and the Challenge questions still needed real thought, that is exactly the shape genuine mastery takes, fast and confident on the routine cases, careful and deliberate on the ones that combine several ideas at once.

CHAPTER 23

Mock Assessment: Comprehensive Review

A third and final full-length assessment, structured the same way as Chapter 22, Foundation questions first, then Clinical Application, then Challenge. Treat this one as a genuine dress rehearsal: time yourself if that helps you gauge readiness, work entirely on paper, and do not turn to the Solutions section until you have committed to every answer.

Question 1 · Foundation (Chapter 4)

A patient is prescribed 600 mg. Tablets are available in 200 mg strength. How many tablets should be given?

Question 2 · Foundation (Chapter 3)

Convert 0.6 mg to micrograms.

Question 3 · Foundation (Chapter 2)

How many grams of drug are contained in 200 mL of a 3% w/v solution?

Question 4 · Foundation (Chapter 5)

A patient is prescribed 150 mg, available as 250 mg in 10 mL. How many mL should be given?

Question 5 · Foundation (Chapter 3)

A patient weighs 12 stone 2 pounds. Convert this to kilograms, to one decimal place.

Question 6 · Foundation (Chapter 4)

A patient is prescribed 350 mg. Both 100 mg and 175 mg tablets are available. What is the most practical combination?

Question 7 · Clinical Application (Chapter 7)

A patient is prescribed 12 mg by injection, supplied as 30 mg in 3 mL. How many mL should be drawn up?

Question 8 · Clinical Application (Chapter 8)

A patient is prescribed a heparin bolus of 6000 units, supplied as 25,000 units in 5 mL. How many mL should be given?

Question 9 · Clinical Application (Chapter 10)

A patient is prescribed 1.5 litres over 12 hours via pump. What rate, in mL per hour, should the pump be set to?

Question 10 · Clinical Application (Chapter 10)

A 400 mL bag is prescribed over 5 hours using a giving set with a drop factor stated on the packaging as 15 drops per mL. What is the rate in drops per minute?

Question 11 · Clinical Application (Chapter 11)

An infusion running at 80 mL per hour from a 500 mL bag has had 240 mL infused. How much longer will it take to complete?

Question 12 · Clinical Application (Chapter 14)

A patient weighing 55 kg is prescribed a drug at 7 mg per kg. What is the total dose required?

Question 13 · Clinical Application (Chapter 16)

A child weighing 19 kg is prescribed a drug at 30 mg per kg per day, in two divided doses. What is the amount for each individual dose?

Question 14 · Clinical Application (Chapter 15)

Calculate the BSA of a patient who is 172 cm tall and weighs 68 kg, using the Mosteller formula.

Question 15 · Challenge (Chapters 12 and 19)

A titrated infusion calculation for a critically unwell patient produces a rate of 0.6 mL per hour, where the drug's usual working range for similarly sized patients is 4 to 8 mL per hour. A colleague, asked for an independent check, arrives at the same 0.6 mL per hour figure by the same method. Is the calculation now confirmed safe to programme?

Question 16 · Challenge (Chapters 14 and 16)

A 33 kg child is prescribed a drug at 25 mg per kg, with a stated maximum single dose of 700 mg. What should happen?

Question 17 · Challenge (Chapter 4)

A calculation for a patient prescribed 150 mg, using a stock strength of 50 mg per tablet, is worked as 50 ÷ 150, giving 0.33. A rough estimate suggested the answer should be around 3 tablets. What is the correct answer?

Question 18 · Challenge (Chapter 8)

A nurse preparing to administer insulin notices that the patient's pre-filled pen is labelled 300 units per mL. The nurse has previously only administered U-100 insulin. What is the most important action before proceeding?

Question 19 · Challenge (Chapter 5 and 7)

A suspension has been sitting unshaken on a shelf for several hours before a dose is drawn up. The calculation for the dose is performed correctly. Is the resulting dose necessarily safe?

Question 20 · Challenge (Chapters 18, 19, and 20)

A nurse is interrupted mid-calculation by an urgent call bell, deals with the patient, and returns several minutes later. Feeling behind on time, they decide to continue from where they believe they left off rather than starting again. What does this book recommend, and why?

Closing Note

That is the last graded assessment in this book. If Chapter 6 felt effortful and this one felt, if not effortless, then at least familiar and manageable, that difference is the entire point of everything between them. The specific numbers in these questions will fade from memory. The reasoning underneath them, dose required against dose available, units checked before anything is calculated, an estimate formed before the precise answer, a result checked against what actually makes clinical sense, is what this book was built to leave you with.

Quick Reference Formula Sheet

Tablets and Capsules

Number of tablets = Dose required ÷ Dose available

Liquid Medications and Injections

Volume to give = (Dose required ÷ Dose available) × Volume the available strength occupies

Percentage Concentration

A percentage solution (percentage weight in volume, % w/v, the most common form) states grams per 100 mL. Amount in a given volume = (percentage ÷ 100) × total volume. Check whether a % v/v or % w/w preparation is involved before assuming this applies.

Ratio Strength

A ratio such as 1:1000 means 1 g in 1000 mL, equivalent to 1 mg per mL. Convert to mg per mL before calculating.

IV Pump Rate

Rate in mL/hour = Total volume (mL) ÷ Total time (hours). Volume = Rate × Time. Time = Volume ÷ Rate.

Drops per Minute (Gravity Infusion)

Drops per minute = (Volume in mL × Drop factor) ÷ Time in minutes. Always convert time to minutes first.

Weight-Based Dosing

Total dose = Dose per kg × Patient weight in kg. If the figure given is a daily dose, divide by the number of doses per day before administering.

Body Surface Area (Mosteller Formula)

BSA (m^2) = square root of [(Height in cm × Weight in kg) ÷ 3600]. Total dose = Dose per m^2 × BSA.

Unit Conversions

1 kg = 1000 g. 1 g = 1000 mg. 1 mg = 1000 micrograms. 1 litre = 1000 mL. 1 kg ≈ 2.2 lb. 1 stone = 14 lb.

Glossary

Dose available: The strength of the medication as supplied, for example the amount in one tablet or in a stated volume of liquid.

Dose required: The amount of a medication that has been prescribed for a patient to receive.

Drop factor: The number of drops delivered by a specific giving set that equal 1 mL, printed on the set's packaging.

Displacement volume: The volume a dissolved powder adds to a diluent during reconstitution, generally already accounted for in manufacturer instructions.

Reconstitution: The process of dissolving a powdered medication in a diluent to form a solution of known concentration before a dose is drawn up.

Titration: Adjusting a medication dose, often an infusion rate, up or down in response to a patient's ongoing clinical measurements.

Unit (drug measurement): A measure of biological activity or potency, used for certain drugs such as insulin and heparin, that cannot be converted to a mass-based measurement such as milligrams.

Body surface area (BSA): An estimate of the total surface area of the body, measured in square metres, used to calculate doses for certain high-risk medications including many chemotherapy agents.

Independent double-check: A second, separate calculation of a dose performed by another person directly from the original prescription, without reference to the first calculation, then compared for agreement.

Dose error reduction software: Software built into many infusion pumps that compares a programmed rate against a preset safe range for a specific drug and alerts if the rate falls outside it.

Further Reading and Resources

This book is intended to build the underlying reasoning behind safe drug calculations, not to replace the specific reference sources you will rely on throughout your career for dosing information, local policy, and drug-specific guidance. Not every calculation in this book needs an academic citation of its own, but the clinical safety claims made throughout it, particularly around insulin, tablet splitting, and checking practices, are grounded in the current guidance and literature listed below, and it is worth being familiar with these sources directly rather than relying on this book as a substitute for them.

Professional Standards

The Nursing and Midwifery Council's Standards of Proficiency for Registered Nurses set the professional framework within which all of the calculation methods in this book are intended to sit, and specifically require accuracy in calculating and administering medicines as part of safe, person-centred care. These have superseded the NMC's former Standards for Medicines Management, and it is the current Standards of Proficiency, alongside the NMC Code, that should be treated as the up to date professional anchor.

It is worth knowing explicitly, and worth revisiting whenever calculation practice feels discouraging, that the NMC's standards for pre-registration nursing programmes require the medicines calculation component of numeracy assessment to be passed at 100%, not merely a comfortable majority. This is not stated to add pressure, but to explain plainly why this subject is treated with the seriousness it is throughout your training, and why a book built around genuine understanding, rather than memorised shortcuts, is worth the additional time it asks of you early on.

Dosing and Medicines Information

The British National Formulary and the British National Formulary for Children remain the standard UK reference for dosing information, maximum doses, and drug-specific cautions, and should always be consulted for current, drug-specific guidance rather than relying on memory or a general calculation method alone.

The NHS Specialist Pharmacy Service publishes practical, regularly updated guidance on specific medicines handling questions, including whether particular tablets can be crushed or capsules opened, and is a reliable first point of reference for exactly the kind of formulation-specific question raised in Chapter 4.

The Royal Pharmaceutical Society publishes broader professional guidance relevant to medicines optimisation and safe administration, complementing the drug-specific detail found in the BNF and BNFC.

Medication Safety Alerts

The Medicines and Healthcare products Regulatory Agency issues drug safety updates that highlight emerging risks with specific medicines, including the guidance on higher-strength insulin products referenced in Chapter 8, and is worth following for exactly the kind of safety-relevant change that a printed book cannot update itself.

NHS England publishes enduring patient safety standards covering medication safety, including guidance on safe abbreviations and labelling practices, several of which, including writing "units" and "micrograms" in full, are reflected directly in this book's own conventions.

Your employing organisation's medicines management policy will set out local requirements for independent double-checking, high-risk medication procedures, and the specific equipment and formulations approved for use in your clinical area, and these local policies take precedence over any general principle discussed in this book where the two differ.

On Mathematics Anxiety and Medication Error

A substantial body of nursing education literature examines the relationship between mathematics anxiety, numeracy confidence, and medication calculation error specifically, distinct from general mathematics education research. Several key studies are listed in full in the reference list below, including McMullan, Jones and Lea's widely cited work establishing the link between anxiety, self-efficacy, and drug calculation ability in British nursing students, and Williams and Davis's scoping review of maths anxiety and dosage calculation errors more broadly. This literature broadly supports the distinction drawn in Chapter 1 of this book between a genuine numeracy skills gap and anxiety-driven underperformance, and is worth exploring further for any reader interested in the evidence behind that distinction, or in supporting students and colleagues who experience it.

Full Reference List

The sources named above are listed here in full for ease of reference. Always check the organisation's own website for the current edition of any of these, since standards, formularies, and safety guidance are updated more frequently than a printed book can reflect.

1. Nursing and Midwifery Council. Standards of Proficiency for Registered Nurses. London: NMC. Available at: nmc.org.uk

2. Nursing and Midwifery Council. Standards for Pre-Registration Nursing Programmes. London: NMC. Available at: nmc.org.uk

3. Nursing and Midwifery Council. The Code: Professional Standards of Practice and Behaviour for Nurses, Midwives and Nursing Associates. London: NMC. Available at: nmc.org.uk

4. Joint Formulary Committee. British National Formulary. London: BMJ Group and Pharmaceutical Press. Available at: bnf.nice.org.uk

5. Joint Formulary Committee. British National Formulary for Children. London: BMJ Group and Pharmaceutical Press. Available at: bnfc.nice.org.uk

6. NHS Specialist Pharmacy Service. Managing the Risk of Confusion Between Insulin Products. Available at: sps.nhs.uk/articles/managing-the-risk-of-confusion-between-insulin-products/

7. NHS Specialist Pharmacy Service. Medicines handling guidance, including advice on crushing tablets and opening capsules. Available at: sps.nhs.uk

8. Medicines and Healthcare products Regulatory Agency. Drug Safety Update: high-strength, fixed-combination and biosimilar insulin products, minimising the risk of medication error. Available at: gov.uk/drug-safety-update

9. Medicines and Healthcare products Regulatory Agency. Drug Safety Update (ongoing monthly series). Available at: gov.uk/drug-safety-update

10. NHS England. Patient Safety Alerts and Enduring Standards: Medication Safety. Available at: england.nhs.uk/patient-safety

11. NHS England. Never Events List. Available at: england.nhs.uk/patient-safety

12. Royal Pharmaceutical Society. Professional guidance on the safe and secure handling of medicines. Available at: rpharms.com

13. Royal College of Nursing. Medicines management guidance for nursing staff. Available at: rcn.org.uk

14. World Health Organization. Global Patient Safety Challenge: Medication Without Harm. Geneva: WHO. Available at: who.int

15. electronic Medicines Compendium (emc). Summary of Product Characteristics for individual licensed medicines, including specific insulin products. Available at: medicines.org.uk/emc

16. Care Quality Commission. Guidance on medicines management for regulated health and social care providers. Available at: cqc.org.uk

17. McMullan, M., Jones, R. and Lea, S. (2012) Math anxiety, self-efficacy, and ability in British undergraduate nursing students. Research in Nursing & Health, 35(2), pp.178-186. https://doi.org/10.1002/nur.21460

18. McMullan, M., Jones, R. and Lea, S. (2010) Patient safety: numerical skills and drug calculation abilities of nursing students and Registered Nurses. Journal of Advanced Nursing, 66(4), pp.891-899. https://doi.org/10.1111/j.1365-2648.2010.05258.x

19. Williams, B. and Davis, S. (2016) Maths anxiety and medication dosage calculation errors: a scoping review. Nurse Education in Practice, 20, pp.139-146. https://doi.org/10.1016/j.nepr.2016.08.005

20. Wright, K. (2010) Do calculation errors by nurses cause medication errors in clinical practice? A literature review. Nurse Education Today, 30(1), pp.85-97. https://doi.org/10.1016/j.nedt.2009.06.009

Solutions

Full worked solutions for every practice set and mock assessment in this book, grouped by chapter. Attempt every question on paper before turning to the relevant section here.

Chapter 6: Practice Set 1: Tablets, Capsules, and Liquid Medications

Question 1 · Foundation

A patient is prescribed 1 g of a drug. Tablets are available in 500 mg strength. How many tablets should be given?

Step 1: Convert units so both quantities match: 1 g = 1000 mg.

Step 2: Dose required: 1000 mg. Dose available: 500 mg per tablet.

Step 3: Divide: 1000 ÷ 500 = 2.

Answer: Give 2 tablets

Question 2 · Foundation

A prescription states 62.5 micrograms. Tablets are available in 0.125 mg strength. How many tablets should be given?

Step 1: Convert both quantities to the same unit. Convert 0.125 mg to micrograms: 0.125 × 1000 = 125 micrograms.

Step 2: Dose required: 62.5 micrograms. Dose available: 125 micrograms per tablet.

Step 3: Divide: 62.5 ÷ 125 = 0.5.

Answer: Half a tablet solves the arithmetic, but do not act on that alone. Check the product information or pharmacy guidance to confirm this specific tablet can be safely divided before administering half.

Question 3 · Foundation

A patient is prescribed 375 mg of a drug, available as a suspension of 125 mg in 5 mL. How many mL should be given?

Step 1: Dose required: 375 mg. Dose available: 125 mg. Volume: 5 mL.

Step 2: Divide: 375 ÷ 125 = 3.

Step 3: Multiply by volume: 3 × 5 mL = 15 mL.

Answer: Give 15 mL

Question 4 · Clinical Application

A patient is prescribed 180 mg of a drug, available as 300 mg in 10 mL. How many mL should be given, rounded to a syringe graduated in 0.1 mL increments?

Step 1: Dose required: 180 mg. Dose available: 300 mg. Volume: 10 mL.

Step 2: Divide: 180 ÷ 300 = 0.6.

Step 3: Multiply by volume: 0.6 × 10 mL = 6 mL.

Step 4: 6 mL is already a measurable increment on the syringe, no further rounding needed.

Answer: Give 6 mL

Question 5 · Clinical Application

How many grams of drug are contained in 40 mL of a 10% solution?

Step 1: A 10% solution contains 10 g per 100 mL.

Step 2: Find the scaling factor for 40 mL: 40 ÷ 100 = 0.4.

Step 3: Multiply: 10 g × 0.4 = 4 g.

Answer: 40 mL contains 4 g

Question 6 · Clinical Application

A drug is supplied as a 1:1000 solution. How many mg are contained in 2 mL?

Step 1: 1:1000 means 1 g in 1000 mL, which is the same as 1 mg per mL.

Step 2: Multiply the concentration by the volume: 1 mg × 2 = 2 mg.

Answer: 2 mL contains 2 mg

Question 7 · Challenge

A patient is prescribed 450 mg of a drug. Tablets are available in both 150 mg and 225 mg strengths. What is the most practical combination?

Step 1: Check 225 mg tablets: 450 ÷ 225 = 2, giving exactly 450 mg with two whole tablets.

Step 2: Check 150 mg tablets: 450 ÷ 150 = 3, requiring three whole tablets.

Step 3: Two tablets is fewer than three, so the 225 mg strength is the more practical choice.

Answer: Give two 225 mg tablets

Question 8 · Challenge

A patient is prescribed 0.6 g of a drug, available as a suspension of 240 mg in 5 mL. How many mL should be given?

Step 1: Convert units to match: 0.6 g = 600 mg.

Step 2: Dose required: 600 mg. Dose available: 240 mg. Volume: 5 mL.

Step 3: Divide: 600 ÷ 240 = 2.5.

Step 4: Multiply by volume: 2.5 × 5 mL = 12.5 mL.

Answer: Give 12.5 mL

Question 9 · Foundation

A patient is prescribed 250 mg of a drug. Tablets are available in 125 mg strength. How many tablets should be given?

Step 1: Dose required: 250 mg. Dose available: 125 mg.

Step 2: Divide: 250 ÷ 125 = 2.

Answer: Give 2 tablets

Question 10 · Foundation

Convert 0.75 g to mg.

Step 1: 1 g = 1000 mg.

Step 2: 0.75 × 1000 = 750.

Answer: 0.75 g = 750 mg

Question 11 · Clinical Application

A patient is prescribed 90 mg of a drug, available as a suspension of 60 mg in 5 mL. How many mL should be given?

Step 1: Dose required: 90 mg. Dose available: 60 mg. Volume: 5 mL.

Step 2: Divide: 90 ÷ 60 = 1.5.

Step 3: Multiply by volume: 1.5 × 5 mL = 7.5 mL.

Answer: Give 7.5 mL

Question 12 · Clinical Application

A patient is prescribed 800 micrograms of a drug. Tablets are available in 0.4 mg strength. How many tablets should be given?

Step 1: Convert 0.4 mg to micrograms: 0.4 × 1000 = 400 micrograms.

Step 2: Dose required: 800 micrograms. Dose available: 400 micrograms.

Step 3: Divide: 800 ÷ 400 = 2.

Answer: Give 2 tablets

Question 13 · Challenge

A patient is prescribed 0.9 g of a drug per day, available as a suspension of 300 mg in 10 mL, to be given in three divided doses. How many mL should be given per dose?

Step 1: Convert 0.9 g to mg: 0.9 × 1000 = 900 mg per day.

Step 2: Divide by number of doses: 900 ÷ 3 = 300 mg per dose.

Step 3: Dose required: 300 mg. Dose available: 300 mg. Volume: 10 mL.

Step 4: Divide: 300 ÷ 300 = 1. Multiply by volume: 1 × 10 mL = 10 mL.

Answer: Give 10 mL per dose, three times a day

Question 14 · Challenge

A calculation for a patient prescribed 600 mg, using a stock strength of 200 mg per tablet, is worked as 200 ÷ 600, giving 0.33. What does this suggest, and what is the correct answer?

Step 1: A dose of 600 mg is larger than a single 200 mg tablet, so the answer should be more than one tablet, not less.

Step 2: An answer of 0.33 conflicts directly with that expectation.

Step 3: The formula was applied backwards. The correct calculation is 600 ÷ 200 = 3.

Answer: The correct answer is 3 tablets. The original working had dose required and dose available reversed.

Chapter 9: Practice Set 2: Injections, Reconstitution, and Unit-Based Dosing

Question 1 · Foundation

A patient is prescribed 15 mg of a drug by subcutaneous injection. It is supplied as 30 mg in 3 mL. How many mL should be given?

Step 1: Dose required: 15 mg. Dose available: 30 mg. Volume: 3 mL.

Step 2: Divide: 15 ÷ 30 = 0.5.

Step 3: Multiply by volume: 0.5 × 3 mL = 1.5 mL.

Answer: Give 1.5 mL

Question 2 · Foundation

A calculation produces a required volume of 0.22 mL. Which syringe is most appropriate: a 1 mL syringe graduated in 0.01 mL, or a 2 mL syringe graduated in 0.1 mL?

Step 1: 0.22 mL requires precision to the nearest 0.01 mL to be measured accurately.

Step 2: A 2 mL syringe graduated in 0.1 mL could only measure to the nearest 0.2 mL, forcing rounding to 0.2 mL.

Step 3: A 1 mL syringe graduated in 0.01 mL can measure 0.22 mL exactly.

Answer: Use the 1 mL syringe graduated in 0.01 mL

Question 3 · Foundation

A powder for injection is reconstituted per the manufacturer's instructions to give a solution of 1 g in 10 mL. A patient is prescribed 400 mg. How many mL should be given?

Step 1: Convert units to match: 1 g = 1000 mg.

Step 2: Dose required: 400 mg. Dose available: 1000 mg. Volume: 10 mL.

Step 3: Divide: 400 ÷ 1000 = 0.4.

Step 4: Multiply by volume: 0.4 × 10 mL = 4 mL.

Answer: Give 4 mL

Question 4 · Clinical Application

A patient is prescribed a heparin bolus of 7500 units. It is supplied as 25,000 units in 5 mL. How many mL should be given?

Step 1: Dose required: 7500 units. Dose available: 25,000 units. Volume: 5 mL.

Step 2: Divide: 7500 ÷ 25,000 = 0.3.

Step 3: Multiply by volume: 0.3 × 5 mL = 1.5 mL.

Answer: Give 1.5 mL

Question 5 · Clinical Application

An insulin infusion is to be prepared at 1 unit per mL using 40 units of insulin made up with sodium chloride 0.9%. What total volume should the insulin be made up to?

Step 1: Target concentration: 1 unit per mL.

Step 2: Total units available: 40 units.

Step 3: At 1 unit per mL, total volume in mL equals total units.

Answer: Make up to a total volume of 40 mL

Question 6 · Clinical Application

A patient is prescribed 300 micrograms of a drug by injection. It is supplied as 0.5 mg in 1 mL. How many mL should be given?

Step 1: Convert units to match: 0.5 mg = 500 micrograms.

Step 2: Dose required: 300 micrograms. Dose available: 500 micrograms. Volume: 1 mL.

Step 3: Divide: 300 ÷ 500 = 0.6.

Step 4: Multiply by volume: 0.6 × 1 mL = 0.6 mL.

Answer: Give 0.6 mL

Question 7 · Challenge

A patient is prescribed 600 mg of a drug by injection. Two vial strengths are available: 300 mg in 2 mL, and 600 mg in 4 mL. Which is the more practical choice, and what volume is drawn up?

Step 1: Using the 300 mg in 2 mL vial: 600 ÷ 300 = 2, then 2 × 2 mL = 4 mL, requiring the full contents of two vials.

Step 2: Using the 600 mg in 4 mL vial: 600 ÷ 600 = 1, then 1 × 4 mL = 4 mL, requiring the full contents of a single vial.

Step 3: Both give the same final volume, but using one 600 mg vial avoids opening a second vial unnecessarily.

Answer: Use the 600 mg in 4 mL vial, draw up 4 mL

Question 8 · Challenge: Spot the Error

A nurse is asked to draw up 12 units of insulin. Finding no insulin syringe available, they draw up 0.12 mL of U-100 insulin using a standard 1 mL syringe, reasoning that the markings can be read directly as units. Is this calculation and approach safe?

Step 1: U-100 insulin contains 100 units per mL, so 12 units corresponds to 12 ÷ 100 = 0.12 mL, which is arithmetically correct.

Step 2: However, a standard 1 mL syringe is not designed or intended for insulin administration, and using it deviates from safe practice regardless of whether the maths is correct.

Step 3: The correct action is to obtain a proper insulin syringe or insulin pen device calibrated directly in units, not to substitute a standard syringe with a converted volume.

Answer: The arithmetic is correct, but the approach is unsafe. Insulin must always be drawn up using a device calibrated in units, never a standard mL syringe, regardless of whether the volume has been calculated correctly.

Question 9 · Foundation

A patient is prescribed 20 mg of a drug by injection, supplied as 40 mg in 2 mL. How many mL should be drawn up?

Step 1: Dose required: 20 mg. Dose available: 40 mg. Volume: 2 mL.

Step 2: Divide: 20 ÷ 40 = 0.5.

Step 3: Multiply by volume: 0.5 × 2 mL = 1 mL.

Answer: Draw up 1 mL

Question 10 · Foundation

A drug is supplied as a 1:10,000 solution. How many mg are in 10 mL?

Step 1: 1:10,000 means 1 g in 10,000 mL, equivalent to 0.1 mg per mL.

Step 2: Multiply: 0.1 mg × 10 = 1 mg.

Answer: 10 mL contains 1 mg

Question 11 · Clinical Application

A patient is prescribed a heparin bolus of 5000 units, supplied as 25,000 units in 5 mL. How many mL should be given?

Step 1: Dose required: 5000 units. Dose available: 25,000 units. Volume: 5 mL.

Step 2: Divide: 5000 ÷ 25,000 = 0.2.

Step 3: Multiply by volume: 0.2 × 5 mL = 1 mL.

Answer: Give 1 mL

Question 12 · Clinical Application

A powder for injection is reconstituted per the manufacturer's instructions to give 250 mg in 2 mL. A patient is prescribed 150 mg. How many mL should be given?

Step 1: Dose required: 150 mg. Dose available: 250 mg. Volume: 2 mL.

Step 2: Divide: 150 ÷ 250 = 0.6.

Step 3: Multiply by volume: 0.6 × 2 mL = 1.2 mL.

Answer: Give 1.2 mL

Question 13 · Challenge

A calculation produces a required volume of 0.18 mL. Two syringes are available: a 1 mL syringe graduated in 0.01 mL, and a 2 mL syringe graduated in 0.1 mL. Which should be used, and why does it matter here specifically?

Step 1: 0.18 mL needs precision to the nearest 0.01 mL to be drawn up accurately as calculated.

Step 2: The 2 mL syringe, graduated only in 0.1 mL, would force rounding to either 0.2 mL, an 11% increase on the intended dose.

Step 3: The 1 mL syringe can measure 0.18 mL exactly.

Answer: Use the 1 mL syringe. The rounding forced by the coarser 2 mL syringe would represent a meaningful proportional error on a dose this small.

Question 14 · Challenge

A nurse checks a heparin vial and finds it labelled 1000 units per mL, having expected the 5000 units per mL strength used on the same ward yesterday. What should the nurse do?

Step 1: Chapter 8 established that heparin, unlike insulin, has no single standardised strength, and the specific concentration must be checked on every vial, every time.

Step 2: Assuming yesterday's strength still applies today would risk a fivefold dosing error if the calculation proceeded on the wrong concentration.

Step 3: The correct response is to use the concentration actually printed on the vial in hand, recalculating the required volume accordingly, not to assume consistency with a previous shift.

Answer: Use the concentration printed on today's vial, 1000 units per mL, and recalculate the required volume from that figure. Never assume a heparin strength carries over from a previous dose or shift.

Chapter 13: Practice Set 3: IV Flow Rates and High-Risk Infusions

Question 1 · Foundation

A patient is prescribed 1.5 litres of fluid over 12 hours via an infusion pump. What rate, in mL per hour, should the pump be set to?

Step 1: Convert the volume to mL: 1.5 litres = 1500 mL.

Step 2: Divide the volume by the time: 1500 ÷ 12.

Step 3: 1500 ÷ 12 = 125.

Answer: Set the pump to 125 mL per hour

Question 2 · Foundation

A 250 mL bag is prescribed over 2 hours, using a standard giving set with a drop factor of 20 drops per mL. What is the rate in drops per minute?

Step 1: Convert the time to minutes: 2 hours × 60 = 120 minutes.

Step 2: Multiply volume by drop factor: 250 × 20 = 5000.

Step 3: Divide by time in minutes: 5000 ÷ 120 = 41.67.

Step 4: Round to the nearest whole drop.

Answer: Set the rate to approximately 42 drops per minute

Question 3 · Foundation

An infusion is running at 100 mL per hour from a 1 litre bag. 350 mL has infused so far. How much longer will it take to complete?

Step 1: Find the volume remaining: 1000 mL – 350 mL = 650 mL.

Step 2: Time equals volume divided by rate: 650 ÷ 100.

Step 3: 650 ÷ 100 = 6.5 hours.

Step 4: Convert 0.5 hours to minutes: 0.5 × 60 = 30 minutes.

Answer: A further 6 hours and 30 minutes

Question 4 · Clinical Application

An infusion started at 09:15 is calculated to run for 4 hours and 45 minutes. What time will it complete?

Step 1: Add the hours: 09:15 + 4 hours = 13:15.

Step 2: Add the minutes: 13:15 + 45 minutes = 14:00.

Answer: The infusion will complete at 14:00

Question 5 · Clinical Application

A pump rate of 60 mL per hour needs to be converted to a gravity infusion using a giving set with a drop factor of 20 drops per mL. What is the equivalent rate in drops per minute?

Step 1: Multiply the hourly volume by the drop factor: 60 × 20 = 1200 drops per hour.

Step 2: Divide by 60 to get drops per minute: 1200 ÷ 60 = 20.

Answer: Set the gravity infusion to 20 drops per minute

Question 6 · Clinical Application

A patient weighing 80 kg is prescribed an infusion at 0.05 micrograms per kg per minute. The bag contains 5 mg in 50 mL. What rate, in mL per hour, should the pump be set to?

Step 1: Dose per minute for this patient: 0.05 × 80 = 4 micrograms per minute.

Step 2: Convert to a dose per hour: 4 × 60 = 240 micrograms per hour.

Step 3: Convert bag concentration to micrograms per mL: 5 mg = 5000 micrograms, 5000 ÷ 50 = 100 micrograms per mL.

Step 4: Divide hourly dose by concentration: 240 ÷ 100 = 2.4.

Answer: Set the pump to 2.4 mL per hour

Question 7 · Challenge

A unit of blood, 300 mL, is prescribed over 2 hours using a blood giving set with a drop factor of 15 drops per mL. What is the rate in drops per minute?

Step 1: Convert time to minutes: 2 hours × 60 = 120 minutes.

Step 2: Multiply volume by drop factor: 300 × 15 = 4500.

Step 3: Divide by time: 4500 ÷ 120 = 37.5.

Step 4: Round to the nearest whole drop.

Answer: Set the rate to approximately 38 drops per minute

Question 8 · Challenge: Evaluate the Situation

A nurse calculates a titrated vasopressor rate and, being confident in the answer, asks a colleague to glance at the number on the pump screen and confirm it looks reasonable before starting the infusion. The colleague agrees it looks fine. Has an appropriate independent double-check taken place?

Step 1: An independent double-check requires the second person to calculate the dose separately from the original prescription, without seeing the first calculation.

Step 2: In this scenario, the colleague only reviewed the final number on the pump screen rather than performing their own independent calculation.

Step 3: This is a passive review, not an independent check, and would not reliably catch an error made in the original calculation, particularly a unit or concentration error made early in the working.

Answer: No. This was not an independent double-check. The colleague should calculate the dose separately from the prescription and compare their own answer, not simply review the number already on the pump.

Question 9 · Foundation

A patient is prescribed 2 litres of fluid over 16 hours via a pump. What rate, in mL per hour, should the pump be set to?

Step 1: Convert to mL: 2 litres = 2000 mL.

Step 2: Divide by time: 2000 ÷ 16 = 125.

Answer: Set the pump to 125 mL per hour

Question 10 · Foundation

An infusion is running at 60 mL per hour. How long will it take to give 180 mL?

Step 1: Time = volume ÷ rate.

Step 2: 180 ÷ 60 = 3.

Answer: 3 hours

Question 11 · Clinical Application

A 200 mL bag is prescribed over 90 minutes using a giving set with a drop factor of 20 drops per mL, as stated on the packaging. What is the rate in drops per minute?

Step 1: Multiply volume by drop factor: 200 × 20 = 4000.

Step 2: Divide by time in minutes: 4000 ÷ 90 = 44.4.

Step 3: Round to the nearest whole drop.

Answer: Set the rate to approximately 44 drops per minute

Question 12 · Clinical Application

An infusion running at 90 mL per hour has had 450 mL infused from a 1 litre bag. What time will it finish if it started at 08:20?

Step 1: Volume remaining: 1000 – 450 = 550 mL.

Step 2: Time remaining: 550 ÷ 90 = 6.11 hours, approximately 6 hours 7 minutes.

Step 3: Add to start time: 08:20 + 6 hours = 14:20, + 7 minutes = 14:27.

Answer: Approximately 14:27

Question 13 · Challenge

A patient weighing 65 kg is prescribed a titrated infusion at 0.08 micrograms per kg per minute. The bag contains 4 mg in 40 mL. What rate, in mL per hour, should the pump be set to?

Step 1: Dose per minute for this patient: 0.08 × 65 = 5.2 micrograms per minute.

Step 2: Convert to per hour: 5.2 × 60 = 312 micrograms per hour.

Step 3: Convert bag concentration: 4 mg = 4000 micrograms, 4000 ÷ 40 = 100 micrograms per mL.

Step 4: Divide: 312 ÷ 100 = 3.12.

Answer: Set the pump to 3.12 mL per hour

Question 14 · Challenge

A calculated titrated infusion rate comes out at 45 mL per hour, where similar patients on this drug typically run at 4 to 6 mL per hour. What should the nurse do before programming the pump?

Step 1: A result roughly ten times the typical range strongly suggests a decimal point or unit conversion error, following the sense-check principle from Chapter 12.

Step 2: Programming the pump on this figure without investigating would risk a substantial overdose if the figure is wrong.

Step 3: The appropriate response is to work back through the calculation, checking units and decimal placement, before programming anything.

Answer: Do not programme the pump yet. Recheck the calculation, paying particular attention to units and decimal points, given how far this result sits from the expected range.

Chapter 17: Practice Set 4: Weight-Based, BSA, and Paediatric Dosing

Question 1 · Foundation

A patient weighing 54 kg is prescribed a drug at 8 mg per kg. What is the total dose required?

Step 1: Identify the dose per kg: 8 mg.

Step 2: Identify the weight: 54 kg.

Step 3: Multiply: 8 × 54 = 432.

Answer: The total dose required is 432 mg

Question 2 · Foundation

A child weighing 14 kg is prescribed a drug at 12 mg per kg, available as a suspension of 250 mg in 5 mL. How many mL should be given?

Step 1: Find the total dose: 12 × 14 = 168 mg.

Step 2: Dose required: 168 mg. Dose available: 250 mg. Volume: 5 mL.

Step 3: Divide: 168 ÷ 250 = 0.672.

Step 4: Multiply by volume: 0.672 × 5 mL = 3.36 mL.

Answer: Give 3.36 mL, rounded to a measurable increment on the syringe used, for example 3.4 mL

Question 3 · Foundation

A child weighing 20 kg is prescribed a drug at 50 mg per kg per day, in four divided doses. What is the amount for each individual dose?

Step 1: Find the total daily dose: 50 × 20 = 1000 mg per day.

Step 2: Divide by the number of doses: 1000 ÷ 4.

Step 3: 1000 ÷ 4 = 250.

Answer: Give 250 mg per dose, four times a day

Question 4 · Clinical Application

Calculate the BSA of a patient who is 160 cm tall and weighs 70 kg, using the Mosteller formula.

Step 1: Multiply height by weight: 160 × 70 = 11,200.

Step 2: Divide by 3600: 11,200 ÷ 3600 = 3.111 (rounded).

Step 3: Take the square root: the square root of 3.111 is approximately 1.76.

Answer: The patient's BSA is approximately 1.76 m^2

Question 5 · Clinical Application

A patient has a BSA of 1.6 m^2 and is prescribed a drug at 75 mg per m^2. What is the total dose required?

Step 1: Identify the dose per m^2: 75 mg.

Step 2: Identify the BSA: 1.6 m^2.

Step 3: Multiply: 75 × 1.6 = 120.

Answer: The total dose required is 120 mg

Question 6 · Clinical Application

A 40 kg adolescent is prescribed a drug at 20 mg per kg, with a stated maximum single dose of 700 mg. What should happen next?

Step 1: Calculate the weight-based dose: 20 × 40 = 800 mg.

Step 2: Compare to the stated maximum of 700 mg.

Step 3: 800 mg exceeds the maximum, which is a signal to stop and check, not to self-adjust and proceed.

Answer: Do not administer 800 mg. Check the prescription and figures, and escalate to the prescriber or pharmacist in line with local policy before any dose is given.

Question 7 · Challenge

A neonate weighing 3.2 kg is prescribed a drug at 4 mg per kg. What is the total dose required, to one decimal place?

Step 1: Identify the dose per kg: 4 mg.

Step 2: Identify the weight: 3.2 kg.

Step 3: Multiply: 4 × 3.2 = 12.8.

Answer: The total dose required is 12.8 mg

Question 8 · Challenge: Evaluate the Situation

A nurse calculates a paediatric dose using a weight recorded on the patient's admission three weeks earlier, reasoning that a young child's weight would not have changed enough in that time to matter. Is this reasoning sound?

Step 1: Chapter 16 established that children's weights can change meaningfully over short periods, more quickly than adult weights typically do.

Step 2: A weight-based calculation is only as accurate as the weight used, regardless of how correctly the arithmetic is performed.

Step 3: Three weeks is long enough, particularly in infants and younger children, for weight change to meaningfully shift a calculated dose.

Answer: No, the reasoning is not sound. The child should be weighed again on the day, using calibrated scales, rather than relying on a three-week-old recorded weight for a weight-based calculation.

Question 9 · Foundation

A patient weighing 48 kg is prescribed a drug at 10 mg per kg. What is the total dose required?

Step 1: Dose per kg: 10 mg. Weight: 48 kg.

Step 2: Multiply: 10 × 48 = 480.

Answer: The total dose required is 480 mg

Question 10 · Foundation

A child weighing 22 kg is prescribed a drug at 15 mg per kg per day, in three divided doses. What is the amount for each individual dose?

Step 1: Total daily dose: 15 × 22 = 330 mg.

Step 2: Divide by number of doses: 330 ÷ 3 = 110.

Answer: Give 110 mg per dose, three times a day

Question 11 · Clinical Application

Calculate the BSA of a patient who is 180 cm tall and weighs 85 kg, using the Mosteller formula.

Step 1: Multiply height by weight: 180 × 85 = 15,300.

Step 2: Divide by 3600: 15,300 ÷ 3600 = 4.25.

Step 3: Square root of 4.25 is approximately 2.06.

Answer: The patient's BSA is approximately 2.06 m^2

Question 12 · Clinical Application

A patient has a BSA of 1.9 m^2 and is prescribed a drug at 60 mg per m^2. What is the total dose required?

Step 1: Dose per m^2: 60 mg. BSA: 1.9 m^2.

Step 2: Multiply: 60 × 1.9 = 114.

Answer: The total dose required is 114 mg

Question 13 · Challenge

A 30 kg child is prescribed a drug at 12 mg per kg, available as a suspension of 250 mg in 5 mL, with a stated maximum single dose of 300 mg. What should happen?

Step 1: Calculate the weight-based dose: 12 × 30 = 360 mg.

Step 2: Compare to the maximum: 360 mg exceeds 300 mg.

Step 3: This is a signal to stop and check, not to proceed with either figure independently.

Answer: Do not administer 360 mg. Check the prescription and figures, and escalate to the prescriber or pharmacist in line with local policy before calculating a volume to give.

Question 14 · Challenge

A nurse is asked to calculate a chemotherapy dose based on BSA and, being confident with the Mosteller formula, works it out by hand rather than using the ward's validated BSA calculator, to save time. What does Chapter 15 say about this approach?

Step 1: Chapter 15 explicitly cautions that BSA-based chemotherapy dosing should be calculated using a validated calculator or nomogram in real practice, not manual arithmetic.

Step 2: This reflects the particularly narrow safety margin and multi-step nature of chemotherapy dosing, where an intermediate error in a hand-calculated BSA compounds into the final dose.

Step 3: Manual calculation is valuable for understanding where the number comes from, but is not a substitute for the validated tool in actual clinical use.

Answer: This approach is not appropriate. The ward's validated BSA calculator should be used for the actual chemotherapy dose, regardless of confidence with the manual formula, given the narrow safety margin involved.

Chapter 21: Mock Assessment: Final Challenge

Question 1 · Foundation (Chapter 4)

A patient is prescribed 900 mg of a drug. Tablets are available in 300 mg strength. How many tablets should be given?

Step 1: Dose required: 900 mg. Dose available: 300 mg.

Step 2: Divide: 900 ÷ 300 = 3.

Answer: Give 3 tablets

Question 2 · Foundation (Chapter 5)

A patient is prescribed 300 mg of a drug, available as 100 mg in 4 mL. How many mL should be given?

Step 1: Dose required: 300 mg. Dose available: 100 mg. Volume: 4 mL.

Step 2: Divide: 300 ÷ 100 = 3.

Step 3: Multiply by volume: 3 × 4 mL = 12 mL.

Answer: Give 12 mL

Question 3 · Foundation (Chapter 3)

A prescription states 0.4 mg. Stock is labelled in micrograms. Convert 0.4 mg to micrograms.

Step 1: 1 mg = 1000 micrograms.

Step 2: 0.4 × 1000 = 400.

Answer: 0.4 mg = 400 micrograms

Question 4 · Foundation (Chapter 7)

A patient is prescribed 60 mg of a drug by injection, supplied as 100 mg in 2 mL. How many mL should be drawn up, and which syringe size is most appropriate?

Step 1: Dose required: 60 mg. Dose available: 100 mg. Volume: 2 mL.

Step 2: Divide: 60 ÷ 100 = 0.6.

Step 3: Multiply by volume: 0.6 × 2 mL = 1.2 mL.

Step 4: 1.2 mL is a small volume best measured on a 2 mL syringe graduated in 0.1 mL, rather than a larger syringe with coarser graduations.

Answer: Draw up 1.2 mL using a 2 mL syringe

Question 5 · Clinical Application (Chapter 8)

A patient is prescribed a heparin bolus of 2000 units, supplied as 5000 units in 5 mL. How many mL should be given?

Step 1: Dose required: 2000 units. Dose available: 5000 units. Volume: 5 mL.

Step 2: Divide: 2000 ÷ 5000 = 0.4.

Step 3: Multiply by volume: 0.4×5 mL = 2 mL.

Answer: Give 2 mL

Question 6 · Clinical Application (Chapter 10)

A patient is prescribed 1.2 litres of fluid over 10 hours via a pump. What rate, in mL per hour, should the pump be set to?

Step 1: Convert to mL: 1.2 litres = 1200 mL.

Step 2: Divide by time: $1200 \div 10 = 120$.

Answer: Set the pump to 120 mL per hour

Question 7 · Clinical Application (Chapter 10)

A 500 mL bag is prescribed over 4 hours using a standard giving set with a drop factor of 20 drops per mL. What is the rate in drops per minute?

Step 1: Convert time to minutes: $4 \times 60 = 240$ minutes.

Step 2: Multiply volume by drop factor: $500 \times 20 = 10{,}000$.

Step 3: Divide by time: $10{,}000 \div 240 = 41.67$.

Step 4: Round to the nearest whole drop.

Answer: Set the rate to approximately 42 drops per minute

Question 8 · Clinical Application (Chapter 11)

An infusion running at 150 mL per hour from a 1 litre bag has had 900 mL infused. How much longer will it take to complete?

Step 1: Volume remaining: $1000 - 900 = 100$ mL.

Step 2: Time = volume ÷ rate: $100 \div 150 = 0.67$ hours.

Step 3: Convert to minutes: $0.67 \times 60 \approx 40$ minutes.

Answer: Approximately 40 minutes remaining

Question 9 · Clinical Application (Chapter 14)

A patient weighing 58 kg is prescribed a drug at 6 mg per kg. What is the total dose required?

Step 1: Dose per kg: 6 mg. Weight: 58 kg.

Step 2: Multiply: $6 \times 58 = 348$.

Answer: The total dose required is 348 mg

Question 10 · Challenge (Chapter 15)

Calculate the BSA of a patient who is 175 cm tall and weighs 80 kg, using the Mosteller formula.

Step 1: Multiply height by weight: 175 × 80 = 14,000.

Step 2: Divide by 3600: 14,000 ÷ 3600 = 3.89 (rounded).

Step 3: Square root of 3.89 is approximately 1.97.

Answer: The patient's BSA is approximately 1.97 m^2

Question 11 · Challenge (Chapter 16)

A 50 kg adolescent is prescribed a drug at 18 mg per kg, with a stated maximum single dose of 800 mg. What should happen next?

Step 1: Calculate the weight-based dose: 18 × 50 = 900 mg.

Step 2: Compare to the maximum: 900 mg exceeds 800 mg.

Step 3: This is a signal to stop and check, not a signal to self-adjust and administer the maximum instead.

Answer: Do not administer 900 mg. Check the prescription and calculation, and escalate to the prescriber or pharmacist in line with local policy before giving any dose.

Question 12 · Challenge (Chapters 18 and 19)

A calculation for a patient prescribed 240 mg, using a stock strength of 80 mg per tablet, is worked as 80 ÷ 240, giving 0.33. A rough estimate suggested the answer should be around 3 tablets. What does this tell you, and what is the correct answer?

Step 1: The precise answer, 0.33, is far from the rough estimate of approximately 3, which is a strong signal that something is wrong.

Step 2: Restating the question in plain language: how many 80 mg tablets are needed to reach 240 mg, a dose considerably larger than one tablet.

Step 3: An answer under 1 conflicts directly with this restated question.

Step 4: The formula was applied backwards. The correct calculation is 240 ÷ 80 = 3.

Answer: The mismatch between the estimate and the precise answer correctly flagged a backwards formula. The correct answer is 3 tablets.

Question 13 · Foundation (Chapter 3)

Convert 2.4 g to mg.

Step 1: 1 g = 1000 mg.

Step 2: 2.4 × 1000 = 2400.

Answer: 2.4 g = 2400 mg

Question 14 · Foundation (Chapter 2)

How many grams of drug are contained in 80 mL of a 2.5% w/v solution?

Step 1: A 2.5% w/v solution contains 2.5 g per 100 mL.

Step 2: Scaling factor for 80 mL: 80 ÷ 100 = 0.8.

Step 3: 2.5 × 0.8 = 2.

Answer: 80 mL contains 2 g

Question 15 · Clinical Application (Chapter 5)

A patient is prescribed 450 mg, available as a suspension of 150 mg in 5 mL. How many mL should be given?

Step 1: Dose required: 450 mg. Dose available: 150 mg. Volume: 5 mL.

Step 2: Divide: 450 ÷ 150 = 3.

Step 3: Multiply by volume: 3 × 5 mL = 15 mL.

Answer: Give 15 mL

Question 16 · Clinical Application (Chapter 7)

A patient is prescribed 45 mg by injection, supplied as 60 mg in 3 mL. How many mL should be drawn up?

Step 1: Dose required: 45 mg. Dose available: 60 mg. Volume: 3 mL.

Step 2: Divide: 45 ÷ 60 = 0.75.

Step 3: Multiply by volume: 0.75 × 3 mL = 2.25 mL.

Answer: Draw up 2.25 mL

Question 17 · Clinical Application (Chapter 11)

An infusion running at 75 mL per hour has had 300 mL infused from a 750 mL bag. How much longer will it take to complete?

Step 1: Volume remaining: 750 − 300 = 450 mL.

Step 2: Time = volume ÷ rate: 450 ÷ 75 = 6 hours.

Answer: 6 hours remaining

Question 18 · Challenge (Chapter 8)

A patient is prescribed a heparin bolus of 1500 units, and the nurse checks the vial, finding it labelled 5000 units in 5 mL. How many mL should be given?

Step 1: Dose required: 1500 units. Dose available: 5000 units. Volume: 5 mL.

Step 2: Divide: 1500 ÷ 5000 = 0.3.

Step 3: Multiply by volume: 0.3 × 5 mL = 1.5 mL.

Answer: Give 1.5 mL

Question 19 · Challenge (Chapters 14 and 16)

A 42 kg child is prescribed a drug at 16 mg per kg, with a stated maximum single dose of 600 mg. What should happen?

Step 1: Calculate the weight-based dose: 16 × 42 = 672 mg.

Step 2: Compare to the maximum: 672 mg exceeds 600 mg.

Step 3: This calls for escalation, not independent substitution of either figure.

Answer: Do not administer 672 mg. Check the prescription and figures, and escalate to the prescriber or pharmacist in line with local policy.

Question 20 · Challenge (Chapters 19 and 20)

Midway through a calculation, a nurse is interrupted by a call bell. On returning, they are unsure whether they had already converted the prescribed dose to mg or not, and the figure in front of them could be read either way. What is the safest next step?

Step 1: Chapter 18 identifies interruption as a recognised risk factor for calculation errors, particularly around resuming a partially completed calculation from memory.

Step 2: Continuing from an uncertain partial calculation risks building on an assumption that may already be wrong.

Step 3: The safest response, per Chapter 20, is to restart the calculation from the original prescription, rather than guessing which stage had been reached.

Answer: Restart the calculation from the original prescription. Do not attempt to guess or reconstruct which step had been reached before the interruption.

Chapter 22: Mock Assessment: Foundation to Challenge

Question 1 · Foundation (Chapter 4)

A patient is prescribed 450 mg. Tablets are available in 150 mg strength. How many tablets should be given?

Step 1: Dose required: 450 mg. Dose available: 150 mg.

Step 2: Divide: 450 ÷ 150 = 3.

Answer: Give 3 tablets

Question 2 · Foundation (Chapter 3)

Convert 1500 micrograms to mg.

Step 1: 1000 micrograms = 1 mg.

Step 2: 1500 ÷ 1000 = 1.5.

Answer: 1500 micrograms = 1.5 mg

Question 3 · Foundation (Chapter 2)

How many grams of drug are contained in 60 mL of a 5% w/v solution?

Step 1: A 5% w/v solution contains 5 g per 100 mL.

Step 2: Scaling factor for 60 mL: 60 ÷ 100 = 0.6.

Step 3: 5 × 0.6 = 3.

Answer: 60 mL contains 3 g

Question 4 · Foundation (Chapter 5)

A patient is prescribed 200 mg, available as 100 mg in 5 mL. How many mL should be given?

Step 1: Dose required: 200 mg. Dose available: 100 mg. Volume: 5 mL.

Step 2: Divide: 200 ÷ 100 = 2.

Step 3: Multiply by volume: 2 × 5 mL = 10 mL.

Answer: Give 10 mL

Question 5 · Foundation (Chapter 3)

A patient weighs 9 stone 6 pounds. Convert this to kilograms, to one decimal place.

Step 1: Convert stones to pounds: 9 × 14 = 126.

Step 2: Add extra pounds: 126 + 6 = 132 pounds.

Step 3: Divide by 2.2: 132 ÷ 2.2 = 60.0.

Answer: 9 stone 6 pounds is approximately 60.0 kg

Question 6 · Clinical Application (Chapter 7)

A patient is prescribed 25 mg by injection, supplied as 50 mg in 2 mL. How many mL should be drawn up?

Step 1: Dose required: 25 mg. Dose available: 50 mg. Volume: 2 mL.

Step 2: Divide: 25 ÷ 50 = 0.5.

Step 3: Multiply by volume: 0.5 × 2 mL = 1 mL.

Answer: Draw up 1 mL

Question 7 · Clinical Application (Chapter 8)

A patient is prescribed a heparin bolus of 3000 units, supplied as 10,000 units in 10 mL. How many mL should be given?

Step 1: Dose required: 3000 units. Dose available: 10,000 units. Volume: 10 mL.

Step 2: Divide: 3000 ÷ 10,000 = 0.3.

Step 3: Multiply by volume: 0.3 × 10 mL = 3 mL.

Answer: Give 3 mL

Question 8 · Clinical Application (Chapter 10)

A patient is prescribed 1 litre over 6 hours via pump. What rate, in mL per hour, should the pump be set to?

Step 1: Convert to mL: 1 litre = 1000 mL.

Step 2: Divide by time: 1000 ÷ 6 = 166.67.

Answer: Set the pump to approximately 167 mL per hour

Question 9 · Clinical Application (Chapter 10)

A 300 mL bag is prescribed over 3 hours using a giving set with a drop factor stated on the packaging as 20 drops per mL. What is the rate in drops per minute?

Step 1: Convert time to minutes: 3 × 60 = 180 minutes.

Step 2: Multiply volume by drop factor: 300 × 20 = 6000.

Step 3: Divide by time: 6000 ÷ 180 = 33.33.

Step 4: Round to the nearest whole drop.

Answer: Set the rate to approximately 33 drops per minute

Question 10 · Clinical Application (Chapter 14)

A patient weighing 70 kg is prescribed a drug at 4 mg per kg. What is the total dose required?

Step 1: Dose per kg: 4 mg. Weight: 70 kg.

Step 2: Multiply: 4 × 70 = 280.

Answer: The total dose required is 280 mg

Question 11 · Clinical Application (Chapter 15)

Calculate the BSA of a patient who is 165 cm tall and weighs 60 kg, using the Mosteller formula.

Step 1: Multiply height by weight: 165 × 60 = 9900.

Step 2: Divide by 3600: 9900 ÷ 3600 = 2.75.

Step 3: Square root of 2.75 is approximately 1.66.

Answer: The patient's BSA is approximately 1.66 m^2

Question 12 · Clinical Application (Chapter 16)

A child weighing 16 kg is prescribed a drug at 25 mg per kg per day, in two divided doses. What is the amount for each individual dose?

Step 1: Total daily dose: 25 × 16 = 400 mg.

Step 2: Divide by number of doses: 400 ÷ 2 = 200.

Answer: Give 200 mg per dose, twice a day

Question 13 · Challenge (Chapters 8 and 12)

A nurse is asked to draw up 8 units of a U-100 insulin. No insulin syringe is available, so they calculate 8 ÷ 100 = 0.08 mL and draw this up using a standard 1 mL syringe. Identify every issue with this approach, not just the arithmetic.

Step 1: The arithmetic is technically consistent with a U-100 concentration: 8 units at 100 units per mL is 0.08 mL.

Step 2: However, this assumes the insulin is definitely U-100 without the nurse having actually checked the product and its concentration, which Chapter 8 identifies as an unsafe assumption given that higher-strength insulins exist.

Step 3: Even if the concentration were confirmed as U-100, using a standard mL syringe instead of a proper insulin syringe or pen is unsafe regardless of the arithmetic, because insulin must always be measured on a device calibrated in units.

Answer: Do not proceed this way. Confirm the specific insulin product and its concentration first, then obtain a proper insulin syringe or pen calibrated in units. A standard mL syringe should not be used for insulin under any circumstances, even with a technically correct manual conversion.

Question 14 · Challenge (Chapters 14 and 16)

A 38 kg child is prescribed a drug at 22 mg per kg, with a stated maximum single dose of 750 mg. The calculated dose exceeds the maximum. What should the nurse do?

Step 1: Calculate the weight-based dose: 22 × 38 = 836 mg.

Step 2: Compare to the maximum: 836 mg exceeds 750 mg.

Step 3: This is a signal to stop and escalate, not a licence to independently give 750 mg instead.

Answer: Do not administer 836 mg, and do not simply substitute 750 mg either. Check the prescription and the figures used, and escalate to the prescriber or pharmacist in line with local policy before any dose is given.

Question 15 · Challenge (Chapters 18 and 19)

A calculation for a patient prescribed 320 mg, using a stock strength of 80 mg per tablet, is worked as 80 ÷ 320, giving 0.25. A rough estimate suggested the answer should be around 4 tablets. What does the mismatch tell you, and what is the correct answer?

Step 1: The precise answer, 0.25, is far from the rough estimate of approximately 4, a strong signal something has gone wrong.

Step 2: Restated in plain language: how many 80 mg tablets are needed to reach 320 mg, a dose considerably larger than one tablet.

Step 3: An answer under 1 directly conflicts with this restated question.

Step 4: The formula was applied backwards. The correct calculation is 320 ÷ 80 = 4.

Answer: The mismatch correctly flagged a backwards formula. The correct answer is 4 tablets.

Question 16 · Foundation (Chapter 3)

Convert 3.6 g to mg.

Step 1: 1 g = 1000 mg.

Step 2: 3.6 × 1000 = 3600.

Answer: 3.6 g = 3600 mg

Question 17 · Foundation (Chapter 2)

How many grams of drug are contained in 150 mL of a 1% w/v solution?

Step 1: A 1% w/v solution contains 1 g per 100 mL.

Step 2: Scaling factor for 150 mL: 150 ÷ 100 = 1.5.

Step 3: 1 × 1.5 = 1.5.

Answer: 150 mL contains 1.5 g

Question 18 · Clinical Application (Chapter 11)

An infusion started at 11:05 is calculated to run for 5 hours and 20 minutes. What time will it complete?

Step 1: Add the hours: 11:05 + 5 hours = 16:05.

Step 2: Add the minutes: 16:05 + 20 minutes = 16:25.

Answer: The infusion will complete at 16:25

Question 19 · Clinical Application (Chapter 7)

A patient is prescribed 8 mg by injection, supplied as 20 mg in 2 mL. How many mL should be drawn up, and which syringe size is most appropriate?

Step 1: Dose required: 8 mg. Dose available: 20 mg. Volume: 2 mL.

Step 2: Divide: 8 ÷ 20 = 0.4.

Step 3: Multiply by volume: 0.4 × 2 mL = 0.8 mL.

Step 4: 0.8 mL is best measured on a 1 mL syringe graduated in 0.01 mL, rather than a larger, coarser syringe.

Answer: Draw up 0.8 mL using a 1 mL syringe

Question 20 · Challenge (Chapters 8 and 16)

A nurse preparing an insulin dose for a child notices the insulin pen is labelled 200 units per mL, having previously only worked with U-100 insulin as an adult nurse. The prescription states the dose in units. What should the nurse do?

Step 1: Chapter 8 establishes that insulin concentration must never be assumed, higher-strength preparations including 200 units per mL exist and are in routine use.

Step 2: Because the prescription and the pen both work directly in units, and the pen is calibrated specifically for its own concentration, the number of units to dial does not change based on the concentration.

Step 3: This is a paediatric patient, so the dose-step increment matters as much as the concentration, some pens step in whole units, some in 2-unit steps, and some paediatric-specific devices step in 0.5-unit increments, and the prescribed dose must be achievable on the specific device in hand.

Step 4: The nurse's task is to confirm the product, the concentration, and the dose-step compatibility of this specific pen for this patient, and to dial the prescribed number of units exactly as written, not to attempt any manual conversion or improvise around a mismatch.

Answer: Confirm the insulin product, concentration, device, and dose-step increment are all correct and compatible for this child. If the prescribed dose is achievable on that device, dial the prescribed number of units directly. Do not perform a manual concentration conversion, and do not improvise if the dose does not fit the device's dose-step increment, check with pharmacy or the prescriber instead.

Chapter 23: Mock Assessment: Comprehensive Review

Question 1 · Foundation (Chapter 4)

A patient is prescribed 600 mg. Tablets are available in 200 mg strength. How many tablets should be given?

Step 1: Dose required: 600 mg. Dose available: 200 mg.

Step 2: Divide: 600 ÷ 200 = 3.

Answer: Give 3 tablets

Question 2 · Foundation (Chapter 3)

Convert 0.6 mg to micrograms.

Step 1: 1 mg = 1000 micrograms.

Step 2: 0.6 × 1000 = 600.

Answer: 0.6 mg = 600 micrograms

Question 3 · Foundation (Chapter 2)

How many grams of drug are contained in 200 mL of a 3% w/v solution?

Step 1: A 3% w/v solution contains 3 g per 100 mL.

Step 2: Scaling factor for 200 mL: 200 ÷ 100 = 2.

Step 3: 3 × 2 = 6.

Answer: 200 mL contains 6 g

Question 4 · Foundation (Chapter 5)

A patient is prescribed 150 mg, available as 250 mg in 10 mL. How many mL should be given?

Step 1: Dose required: 150 mg. Dose available: 250 mg. Volume: 10 mL.

Step 2: Divide: 150 ÷ 250 = 0.6.

Step 3: Multiply by volume: 0.6 × 10 mL = 6 mL.

Answer: Give 6 mL

Question 5 · Foundation (Chapter 3)

A patient weighs 12 stone 2 pounds. Convert this to kilograms, to one decimal place.

Step 1: Convert stones to pounds: 12 × 14 = 168.

Step 2: Add extra pounds: 168 + 2 = 170 pounds.

Step 3: Divide by 2.2: 170 ÷ 2.2 = 77.3.

Answer: 12 stone 2 pounds is approximately 77.3 kg

Question 6 · Foundation (Chapter 4)

A patient is prescribed 350 mg. Both 100 mg and 175 mg tablets are available. What is the most practical combination?

Step 1: Using 175 mg tablets: 350 ÷ 175 = 2, two whole tablets.

Step 2: Using 100 mg tablets: 350 ÷ 100 = 3.5, requiring a split tablet.

Step 3: Two whole 175 mg tablets is more practical than three and a half 100 mg tablets.

Answer: Give two 175 mg tablets

Question 7 · Clinical Application (Chapter 7)

A patient is prescribed 12 mg by injection, supplied as 30 mg in 3 mL. How many mL should be drawn up?

Step 1: Dose required: 12 mg. Dose available: 30 mg. Volume: 3 mL.

Step 2: Divide: 12 ÷ 30 = 0.4.

Step 3: Multiply by volume: 0.4 × 3 mL = 1.2 mL.

Answer: Draw up 1.2 mL

Question 8 · Clinical Application (Chapter 8)

A patient is prescribed a heparin bolus of 6000 units, supplied as 25,000 units in 5 mL. How many mL should be given?

Step 1: Dose required: 6000 units. Dose available: 25,000 units. Volume: 5 mL.

Step 2: Divide: 6000 ÷ 25,000 = 0.24.

Step 3: Multiply by volume: 0.24 × 5 mL = 1.2 mL.

Answer: Give 1.2 mL

Question 9 · Clinical Application (Chapter 10)

A patient is prescribed 1.5 litres over 12 hours via pump. What rate, in mL per hour, should the pump be set to?

Step 1: Convert to mL: 1.5 litres = 1500 mL.

Step 2: Divide by time: 1500 ÷ 12 = 125.

Answer: Set the pump to 125 mL per hour

Question 10 · Clinical Application (Chapter 10)

A 400 mL bag is prescribed over 5 hours using a giving set with a drop factor stated on the packaging as 15 drops per mL. What is the rate in drops per minute?

Step 1: Convert time to minutes: 5 × 60 = 300 minutes.

Step 2: Multiply volume by drop factor: 400 × 15 = 6000.

Step 3: Divide by time: 6000 ÷ 300 = 20.

Answer: Set the rate to 20 drops per minute

Question 11 · Clinical Application (Chapter 11)

An infusion running at 80 mL per hour from a 500 mL bag has had 240 mL infused. How much longer will it take to complete?

Step 1: Volume remaining: 500 − 240 = 260 mL.

Step 2: Time = volume ÷ rate: 260 ÷ 80 = 3.25 hours.

Step 3: Convert 0.25 hours to minutes: 0.25 × 60 = 15 minutes.

Answer: A further 3 hours and 15 minutes

Question 12 · Clinical Application (Chapter 14)

A patient weighing 55 kg is prescribed a drug at 7 mg per kg. What is the total dose required?

Step 1: Dose per kg: 7 mg. Weight: 55 kg.

Step 2: Multiply: 7 × 55 = 385.

Answer: The total dose required is 385 mg

Question 13 · Clinical Application (Chapter 16)

A child weighing 19 kg is prescribed a drug at 30 mg per kg per day, in two divided doses. What is the amount for each individual dose?

Step 1: Total daily dose: 30 × 19 = 570 mg.

Step 2: Divide by number of doses: 570 ÷ 2 = 285.

Answer: Give 285 mg per dose, twice a day

Question 14 · Clinical Application (Chapter 15)

Calculate the BSA of a patient who is 172 cm tall and weighs 68 kg, using the Mosteller formula.

Step 1: Multiply height by weight: 172 × 68 = 11,696.

Step 2: Divide by 3600: 11,696 ÷ 3600 = 3.25.

Step 3: Square root of 3.25 is approximately 1.80.

Answer: The patient's BSA is approximately 1.80 m^2

Question 15 · Challenge (Chapters 12 and 19)

A titrated infusion calculation for a critically unwell patient produces a rate of 0.6 mL per hour, where the drug's usual working range for similarly sized patients is 4 to 8 mL per hour. A colleague, asked for an independent check, arrives at the same 0.6 mL per hour figure by the same method. Is the calculation now confirmed safe to programme?

Step 1: Both calculations agreeing is reassuring, but Chapter 19 notes that two people using the identical method and the identical starting assumption can both make the same error, particularly a shared misreading of the prescription or a shared unit mistake.

Step 2: The result sits far outside the expected working range for this drug and patient size, which per Chapter 12 is itself a strong signal to pause regardless of the double-check.

Step 3: The safest next step is to recheck the original prescription and the figures both nurses started from, not simply to trust that agreement between two calculations settles the matter.

Answer: Not necessarily. Two independent calculations agreeing is reassuring but does not rule out a shared error in reading the prescription. Given how far this result sits from the expected range, recheck the original prescription and source figures before programming the pump.

Question 16 · Challenge (Chapters 14 and 16)

A 33 kg child is prescribed a drug at 25 mg per kg, with a stated maximum single dose of 700 mg. What should happen?

Step 1: Calculate the weight-based dose: 25 × 33 = 825 mg.

Step 2: Compare to the maximum: 825 mg exceeds 700 mg.

Step 3: This is a signal to stop and escalate, not to independently give either figure.

Answer: Do not administer 825 mg. Check the prescription and figures, and escalate to the prescriber or pharmacist in line with local policy before any dose is given.

Question 17 · Challenge (Chapter 4)

A calculation for a patient prescribed 150 mg, using a stock strength of 50 mg per tablet, is worked as 50 ÷ 150, giving 0.33. A rough estimate suggested the answer should be around 3 tablets. What is the correct answer?

Step 1: The precise answer, 0.33, conflicts sharply with the rough estimate of approximately 3.

Step 2: Restated in plain language: how many 50 mg tablets are needed to reach 150 mg, a dose larger than one tablet.

Step 3: The formula was applied backwards. The correct calculation is 150 ÷ 50 = 3.

Answer: The correct answer is 3 tablets.

Question 18 · Challenge (Chapter 8)

A nurse preparing to administer insulin notices that the patient's pre-filled pen is labelled 300 units per mL. The nurse has previously only administered U-100 insulin. What is the most important action before proceeding?

Step 1: Chapter 8 warns specifically against assuming a familiar concentration, and 300 units per mL is one of the higher-strength preparations in routine use, supplied as a pre-filled pen rather than a vial.

Step 2: Because the pen is calibrated to dial and deliver the prescribed number of units directly, regardless of the concentration inside it, no manual conversion is needed or appropriate here.

Step 3: The risk lies not in the arithmetic but in treating this pen as interchangeable with a syringe-drawn U-100 dose, including any attempt to withdraw the insulin from the pen into a separate syringe.

Answer: Confirm that the prescribed insulin, its concentration, and the pen are correct for this patient, then dial and deliver the prescribed number of units directly on the pen. Do not withdraw the insulin from the pen into a syringe, and do not attempt a manual concentration conversion.

Question 19 · Challenge (Chapter 5 and 7)

A suspension has been sitting unshaken on a shelf for several hours before a dose is drawn up. The calculation for the dose is performed correctly. Is the resulting dose necessarily safe?

Step 1: Chapter 5 explains that an unshaken suspension can have drug particles unevenly distributed, meaning the concentration at any given point may not match the label.

Step 2: A calculation performed correctly, based on the labelled concentration, assumes that concentration is actually present in the liquid drawn up.

Step 3: If the suspension was not shaken immediately before measuring, the actual dose delivered may not match the calculated one, regardless of how correct the arithmetic was.

Answer: Not necessarily. The suspension should be shaken thoroughly immediately before measuring, regardless of how correct the calculation is, or the concentration actually drawn up may not match the label.

Question 20 · Challenge (Chapters 18, 19, and 20)

A nurse is interrupted mid-calculation by an urgent call bell, deals with the patient, and returns several minutes later. Feeling behind on time, they decide to continue from where they believe they left off rather than starting again. What does this book recommend, and why?

Step 1: Chapter 18 identifies interruption as a well-recognised risk factor for calculation errors, specifically around resuming a partially completed calculation from memory.

Step 2: Chapter 20 recommends restarting the calculation from the original prescription after an interruption, rather than attempting to reconstruct which step had been reached.

Step 3: Feeling time pressure is exactly the condition under which this shortcut becomes tempting and exactly when the risk of an undetected error is highest.

Answer: Restart the calculation from the original prescription rather than continuing from an uncertain partial working. The time pressure that makes this feel inconvenient is exactly why the risk is real.